Cocaine:
Clinical and Biobehavioral Aspects

EDITED BY

Seymour Fisher
The University of Texas Medical Branch at Galveston

Allen Raskin
Wayne State University

E. H. Uhlenhuth
The University of New Mexico

New York   Oxford
OXFORD UNIVERSITY PRESS
1987

Oxford University Press

Oxford   New York   Toronto
Delhi   Bombay   Calcutta   Madras   Karachi
Petaling Jaya   Singapore   Hong Kong   Tokyo
Nairobi   Dar es Salaam   Cape Town
Melbourne   Auckland
and associated companies in
Beirut   Berlin   Ibadan   Nicosia

Library of Congress Cataloging-in-Publication Data
American College of Neuropsychopharmacology.
    Meeting (23rd : 1984 : San Juan, P.R.)
    Cocaine : clinical and biobehavioral aspects.
    "Selected papers from the 23rd annual scientific
meeting of the American College of Neuropsychopharma-
cology (ANCP), December 1984."
    Includes bibliographies and indexes.
    1. Cocaine habit—Congresses. 2. Cocaine—
Physiological effects—Congresses. 3. Cocaine—
Psychological aspects—Congresses. I. Fisher,
Seymour.   II. Raskin, Allen.   III. Uhlenhuth,
E. H. IV. Title. [DNLM: 1. Behavior—drug effects—
congresses. 2. Cocaine—pharmacodynamics—congresses.
3. Substance Abuse—therapy—congresses.
W3 AM312 23rd 1984c / QV 113 A512 1984c]
RC568.C6A47   1984   616.86'3   86-857
ISBN 0-19-504068-6

9 8 7 6 5 4 3 2 1
Printed in the United States of America
on acid-free paper

Preface

Little did Sigmund Freud realize what his experiments with cocaine in the early 1880s, contributing to Koller's 1884 discovery of cocaine-induced local anesthesia, would lead to in the 1980s. As late as 1970, in the fourth edition of Goodman and Gilman's *The Pharmacological Basis of Therapeutics*[1], Jaffe could write "Cocaine abuse is now uncommon in Western countries, although the chewing of coca leaves is still common among the Peruvian Indians of the Andes" (p. 294); and when cocaine abuse did occur in the United States, it was mainly via intraveneous injection and was restricted to a relatively small segment of society.

Now we are faced with a "Coke is it!" (New or Classic) zeitgeist where cocaine use, in all forms, is so widespread as to be a major public health problem. Compounding the problem is the ease with which synthetic "designer" drugs with euphoriant properties can hit the streets. One recent example is that of MDMA (3,4-methyl-enedioxymethamphetamine), often referred to as "Ecstasy." As of July 1, 1985—despite protests from a small group of adherents who believe the drug may have great therapeutic potential—the drug was banned (i.e., labeled with a one-year emergency Schedule I controlled-substance classification) by the U.S. Drug Enforcement Agency as a "serious health threat." And even more recently, we have "crack," the deadliest form of cocaine, making its appearance. With the extensively publicized deaths of two nationally prominent, young, talented athletes in June 1986, the perception of cocaine as a safe drug for recreational or therapeutic use must be clearly labeled as delusional.

In a troubled society, rhetoric may at times play an important role in focusing upon critical social issues, but rhetoric alone cannot provide the solutions to those problems. Ultimately, good decisions regarding systematic actions and governmental interventions can come only from a Solomonic combination of rational thought and sound empirical findings. The presentations selected from the annual meeting of the American College of Neuropsychopharmacology (ACNP) for inclusion in *Cocaine: Clinical and Biobehavioral Aspects* make exceptionally clear the complexity of the problems and the necessity for major innovative research endeavors, both basic and clinical. The possibilities of simple and ready solutions do not appear to be immediate. However, potentially productive and rewarding avenues for multidisciplinary approaches are suggested in many of the chapters. This is of particular importance today, when there are frequent demands for instant results, with pressures to reduce public support for scientific investigation in favor of increased hyperpunitive law-enforcement strategies.

Not since 1972, when opiate addiction was becoming pandemic, has the ACNP devoted a major portion of its annual scientific meeting to a substance abuse theme[2]. For the 1984 meeting the College again attempted to look at a current public health substance abuse problem for the neuropsychopharmacological point of view—that is, ranging from basic neurochemistry and neurophysiology through sociological and anthropological observations to clinical applications. These papers formed the basis for this volume.

A brief review of the content of each chapter will illustrate the range and diversity of clinical and research findings on cocaine contained in this book. The first chapter, by Robert Byck, provides three overviews or three "faces" of cocaine: first, a romantic tale spiced with glowing accounts of its curative powers by luminaries such as Sigmund Freud; second, the history of cocaine as seen from reports in the media, with special attention paid to distortions and biased underplaying of cocaine's harmful effects; and finally a more balanced account of the history of cocaine use and its chemical, clinical, and addictive properties.

In Chapter 2, James Woods and his co-authors examine the behavioral and neuronal actions of cocaine that could account for its abuse potential or, more specifically, its tendency to be self-administered. Based on work with animals, they postulate that the abuse of this drug could arise from its capacity to maintain and increase certain behaviors (its reinforcing effect), and its effects on subjective states, such as feelings of increased well-being, euphoria, increased energy, and decreased fatigue (its discriminative effects). This model has implications for the treatment of cocaine abusers. For example, the authors describe drugs that modify the discriminative effects of cocaine as well as drugs that modify cocaine-reinforced responding. The value of these drugs, primarily dopamine receptor agonists, in the treatment of cocaine abuse is discussed.

Kornetsky and Bain, in Chapter 3, continue the dialogue that Woods and associates started by presenting evidence that the primary basis for the abuse of opiates, as well as cocaine and central nervous system stimulants, is their hedonic or rewarding effect mediated by areas of the brain that subserve intracranial self-stimulation (ICSS). They note that all opioids that are abused, as well as cocaine, lower the threshold for rewarding electrical stimulation in the rat. With regard to treatment implications for cocaine abuse, they state that naloxone blocks this effect, suggesting that this animal model may serve as a basis for testing drugs that could be used to treat cocaine abusers. On the basis of their own work and similiar work on the ICSS model that targeted certain brain sites, Kornetsky and Bain conclude by suggesting that the common neuronal basis for the euphorigenic action of these drugs involves a catecholaminergic and opioid receptor interaction.

The issue of neural substrates for opioid activation and reinforcement that Kornetsky and Bain raise at the end of their chapter is the major theme of Chapter 4, by Koob and his co-authors. Using a model of self-administration of either heroin or cocaine, the authors tested different doses of a number of compounds that block dopamine receptors to see their selective effects on self-administration of heroin or cocaine. On the basis of these and related studies, the authors concluded that the neurochemical substrates responsible for the activating and reinforcing properties of heroin are at one level independent of the midbrain dopamine systems, but that of the nucleus accumbens and its connections play a key role in the neurobiology of opiate reinforcement and activation.

The issue of sensitization to chronic or long-term use of cocaine and possible underlying mechanisms for this phenomenon is the theme of Chapter 5, by Robert Post and colleagues. Whereas tolerance to acute cocaine administration may develop with repeated administration after intervals of minutes to hours, there is now a substantial body of evidence (reviewed in this chapter) that there may be a sensitization or reverse tolerance to many effects of cocaine when administered chronically at longer intervals. The authors suggest that sensitization to chronic use of cocaine can lead to a kindling-like mechanism with the potential for spontaneous seizures. There is also some evidence that lithium may be effective in inhibiting cocaine-induced behavioral sensitization. Although much of this work is preliminary, it has important implications in the treatment of chronic cocaine abusers.

Chapter 6, by Gawin and Kleber, concerns the quality of the research that has been conducted on drug and psychosocial treatment of cocaine abusers. At the outset these authors state that there are as yet no definitive treatments for cocaine abusers. There is also the implication in this chapter that failure to adequately define samples of cocaine abusers and other methodologic flaws may be at least partially responsible for the inability to show treatment effects. For example, they cite differences among cocaine abusers in frequency of use, dosage, route of administration, degree of psychosocial disruption, and so on, as factors that must be considered or controlled when one conducts treatment assessment studies with these individuals. Their review of studies of both psychosocial and pharmacologic treatments for cocaine abusers focuses on methodologic deficiencies in these studies. In highlighting these deficiencies, the authors make a plea for additional well-controlled studies that will provide better answers than are now available on treating cocaine abusers.

Whereas Gawin and Kleber are primarily concerned with research issues in treatment assessment studies, Thomas Crowley (Chapter 7) is concerned with practical issues facing the clinician in the treatment of cocaine abusers. Crowley begins his chapter with a case history of severe cocaine abuse that he uses to illustrate the predisposing factors, signs, symptoms, and course of this disorder. Crowley also reviews currently available information on the treatment of cocaine overdose and recent treatment outcome reports for cocaine abuse. He concludes with a comment shared by a number of other chapter authors that the absence of controlled and well-designed studies precludes any recommendations for one treatment over another at the present time.

The final chapter, by Richard Schultes (Chapter 8), is a scholarly presentation of the magical/religious roles that coca and other new world psychoactive drugs play in primitive societies. Professor Schultes is Director of the Botanical Museum at Harvard University and much of the material in this chapter is drawn from his own experiences as an observer and occasional participant observer of the effects of a variety of new world psychoactive plants on members of primitive tribes. This chapter will have obvious appeal to those with an interest in ethnopsychopharmacology, but it also provides the anthropologist, sociologist, psychologist, and psychiatrist with insights into the key role that psychoactive substances have played and continue to play in some primitive societies. These drugs are used as energizers, in religious ceremonies, to relieve pain, and to escape the "intolerable clutch of reality." It does not take much imagination to find similiar roles for these drugs in "civilized societies."

Having provided a synopsis or overview of the book, we would like to conclude with the hope this volume will stimulate and encourage further thought and research on the problems of cocaine abuse.

We are particularly grateful to Mrs. Delva Siemsen from the University of Texas Medical Branch at Galveston for her editorial assistance along with her intelligence and tenacity in working with the editors and contributors.

January 1986   S. F.
                                  A. R.
                                  E. H. U.

[1]Jaffe, J. H. Drug addiction and drug abuse. In Goodman, L.S., Gilman, A. (eds.), *The Pharmacological Basis of Therapeutics*, 4th edition. New York: Macmillan, 1970, pp. 276–313.
[2]Fisher, S., Freedman, A. F. *Opiate Addiction: Origins and Treatment.* Washington, D.C.: V.H. Winston & Sons, 1974.

Acknowledgments

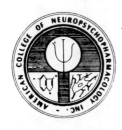

PUBLISHED UNDER THE IMPRIMATUR

OF THE

AMERICAN COLLEGE

OF NEUROPSYCHOPHARMACOLOGY

Many people were very helpful in planning and organizing the American College of Neuropsychopharmacology's 23rd annual plenary session on which this book is based. We are especially grateful to members of the 1984 ACNP Program & Scientific Communications Committee—Chris-Ellyn Johanson, Ph.D., Jack Peter Green, M.D., Ph.D., Israel Hanin, Ph.D., David Segal, Ph.D., Benjamin Bunney, M.D., Dennis Murphy, M.D., Earl Usdin, Ph.D., Michael Goldstein, Ph.D., Arthur Rifkin, M.D., Paul Wender, M. D., Richard Marcus, Ph.D., and Herbert Meltzer, M.D.—and its Publications Committee—Allen Raskin, Ph.D., Monte Buchsbaum, M.D., Elliot Gershon, M.D., Jonathan Cole, M.D., Donald Robinson, M.D., Lewis Seiden, Ph.D., and Menek Goldstein, Ph.D.

Seymour Fisher, Ph.D., *President*
Allen Raskin, Ph.D., *Chairman*
Publications Committee
E.H. Uhlenhuth, M.D., *Chairman*
Program & Scientific
Communications Committee

Contents

Cocaine

1 | Cocaine Use and Research: Three Histories

ROBERT BYCK

THIS chapter was conceived near the end of 1984. It is one hundred years since the publication of Freud's *Über Coca* and one hundred years since the discovery of local anesthesia with cocaine. It is now ten years since the National Institute of Drug Abuse requested proposals to study the human pharmacology of cocaine. Most significantly, it is the year of Orwell's 1984, of doublespeak, of newspeak and of doublethink. Though this chapter is presented in oldspeak, with some use of Orwell's C language, the story of cocaine is rich in doublethink.

Cocaine must be considered in context. It is a plant alkaloid. It is a ritual substance used by twelve million people. It is a local anesthetic of considerable value in medicine. It is a drug of interest to pharmacologists because it is a prototype euphoriant. It is a major drug of abuse associated with robbery, violence, and murder. It is an important commodity whose trade affects the politics of the Americas.

As a commodity cocaine must be considered in economic terms that may have little to do with either its status as a drug of abuse or its prosaic qualities as a natural alkaloid with pharmacological actions. As a commodity it is subject to advertising distortions and a newsworthiness that can influence political processes and public perceptions. Cocaine has become a metaphor for money, power, prestige, and celebrity—as well as either organized crime or white-collar "victimless" crime. There does not seem to be a requirement for precision of statement or substantiation of information when cocaine is described in its metaphorical sense.

The romance of cocaine has started to wear thin. Close to the

3

100th anniversary of the discovery of local anesthesia, this wonder drug's public image is once again on the decline. History repeats itself, even pharmacological history. The drug itself has remained alkaloidal and stable throughout but its image continues to change. Our knowledge of the effects of this substance has not increased markedly since the early part of the century. We may have some early clues and theories about mechanisms but we still do not know the answer to the *real* question about cocaine: Why is it such an attractive and entrapping euphoriant? What is the answer to the mystery of its allure?

I will consider the history of scientific and pharmacological knowledge of cocaine effects in humans against the background of popular images and public perception. A critique of the media interpretation of cocaine-related "news" is important in understanding how public perceptions come about. There is an abundance of material on cocaine, and a rich collection of historical reviews and sources (see, for example, Aldrich & Barker, 1976; Ashley, 1975; Byck, 1974; Grinspoon & Bakalar, 1976; Holmstedt & Fredga, 1981; Liljestrand, 1963, 1967; Martin, 1970; Mortimer, 1901; Musto, 1973; and Petersen 1977.) The mythology of cocaine can, however, warp both the history and the pharmacology. The drug stimulates writers to hyperbole and, judging from the popular press, cocaine sells both magazines and newspapers.

To appreciate and judge any information about cocaine, a reader must be aware of certain facts. The intensity, and sometimes the nature, of cocaine's effects are governed by (1) the form of the drug: natural leaf, cocaine hydrochloride, cocaine paste, or alkaloidal cocaine (free base); (2) the route of administration: oral, intranasal, intravenous, smoked; (3) the dose of the drug; and (4) the timing, as well as the chronocity of the dosage. The perceived and observed effects are modulated by the biological and social characteristics of the individual, as well as the set and setting. For example, when coca leaf is chewed, appreciable blood levels of cocaine are found. This demonstrates both that cocaine is effective by the oral route and that coca chewers are *de facto* users. Nevertheless, a Quechua chewing coca in Cuzco is not the same as a movie star free-basing in Malibu. The drug is a constant but the cultural environment, route, and form are all different.

The oft-repeated and typical recounting of the cocaine legend presents an almost magical and thus attractive background for the drug's use. A history of cocaine as a commodity and a metaphor might be presented as follows.

THE ROMANCE OF COCAINE

A mysterious gift of the gods used in ancient burials, deified in a great civilization of the new world, the leaves of this evergreen shrub made possible the incredible feats of the runners in the highlands of the Inca empire. Noticed by the early explorers, its use was at first reviled as a pagan habit. Its virtues soon became apparent to the Conquistadors, who forced superhuman labors from the oppressed natives with the aid of the stimulant. As both a god and a currency coca was a major influence in the civilization of South America. Brought to Europe as one of many miraculous substances from the new world, it was lauded by scientists and travelers. When the brilliant neuropathologist Sigmund Freud summarized and exalted the substance it came into wide use as a panacea. He used the drug and experimented with it. His *Interpretation of Dreams* and the later development of psychoanalytic method may have been aided by cocaine. Widely utilized as a cure for the morphine and alcohol habits, cocaine was also discovered to be a local anesthetic and so a boon to humanity. It was used by a panoply of the greatest minds of the 19th century. Almost all of those who wrote of cocaine became its victims. Halsted of Johns Hopkins, a man whose silk shirts were laundered in Paris, both discovered nerve block anesthesia and became a cocaine addict. Kings, artists, popes, and presidents extolled the virtues of coca wine (Helfand, 1980) and even the Surgeon General of the Army, William Hammond, endorsed the virtues of the wonder drug. Although public perceptions changed, the drug was widely distributed in elixirs and magical drinks such as Coca-Cola. This material, "the intellectual beverage," still keeps the image and the name before the public. "Coke is it" may be a soft drink advertisement but unauthorized T-shirts relate it to "the real thing."

Yellow journalism thrived on the drug menace. Fear of cocaine-crazed Negroes in the early 20th century South created another irresistible media lure (*New York Herald*, 1913). Cocaine, which fueled the Inca empire, now made bullet-proof blacks. The fear of drugged minorities is a commonality when forces are marshalled to create a public response (Musto, 1973). In the mid-20th century cocaine was news again with stories of its increasing expense, its use by the famous, and an inevitable association with class and influence. In the late 1970s its use by championship athletes associated it with manliness and power. Popular articles described it as the champagne or caviar of drugs. What other white powder could appear on the covers of *Time, Newsweek,* and *TV Guide? The Reader's Digest* headlined it and a local anesthetic became the powdery star of the media.

This presentation, condensed but true in its particulars, can only be construed as an advertisement. Cocaine makes good copy.

DISTORTIONS IN WRITING ABOUT COCAINE

Popular opinion varies between extremes. There seems to be no place for cocaine in the middle—an effective local anesthetic with a relatively great safety margin as such and an effective central stimulant with a high abuse potential. When a nonpolar view is advanced, advocates of the extremes take selected material out of context for public presentation (see, for instance, O'Toole, 1982). Data and history are often selected to make the drug seem irresistible or terrifying. Popular presentations may reflect political biases. For example, in a piece on the Cuban revolutionary Che Guevara, "they saw how the Indians of the Peruvian *Altiplano* (high plateau), whose ancestors were the great Incas, are exploited and brutalized because of their addiction to *coca*" (Harris, 1971) or, in contrast, from a Peruvian scientist supportive of indigenous coca use, "Without adequate scientific evidence it is rather simple to blame coca and the indians who use it for the poverty and backwardness found in the Peruvian Andes" (Cabieses, 1975). The variable quality or pertinence of research is rarely examined and the short presentations demanded by modern media lead to high selectivity. Selection of material for television can even more effectively glorify or damn the drug. For example, the following completely misleading report was presented in Los Angeles on KHJTV (see Notes at the end of the chapter).

> Cocaine may actually be no more harmful to your health than smoking cigarettes or drinking alcohol[1], at least that's according to a six year study of cocaine use[2]. It concludes that the drug is relatively safe[3] and if not taken in large amounts it is not addictive[4]. The study appears in the new issue of *Scientific American.*

The newswriter, basing his material on a widely circulated magazine article (Van Dyke & Byck, 1982) managed four serious distortions in just fifteen seconds.[1]

There may be pious statements about damages or liabilities of cocaine but often the graphics and the mode of presentation make the drug seem worth the risk. *Time* magazine showed a champagne glass full of sparkling white powder on its cover in July 1981 with the headline "HIGH ON COCAINE—a drug with status—and menace." The questionable warning is totally offset by the brilliant graphics. In the text cocaine was referred to as an "all-American drug." the "scientific" explanation was headlined "A fire in the brain"; nerve cells were described as a "string of firecrackers." The net effect of this article was to present a positive and alluring image.

New York magazine (1978) showed a woman snorting through a hundred dollar bill from a sea of white powder. Inside, "the drug of choice" was described by "experts" as "every bit as enjoyable as Freud claimed. There can be no denying that this kind of attention has contributed to the widespread public interest on cocaine. *The New York Times* has characterized the trend toward increasing tolerance of illegal drugs as a "basic paradox in social attitudes towards drugs" (Collins, 1983). And the intensity of interest is no longer confined to users. The commodity is clearly of greater interest than the drug—murders, revolutions, big money, and celebrities are the stuff of popular journalism—and so distortions with no scientific basis are broadcast.

The scientist working on cocaine is inevitably in the public spotlight. It is hard to resist the requests for opinion and information and hard to take the results. Misinterpretations are common and misquotations are standard. Why is this so? Prejudice based on reporter's habits or biases are often overlooked in straight news reporting. We must be particularly concerned if *Time*, *The New York Times*, and *High Times* all agree. For a while they were together in implicitly or explicitly encouraging cocaine use.

Without inquiring into the varied motivations of individual journals and journalists, one can point out that reporting is only as good as its sources. Many "experts" are biased in their advocacy of either the safety or danger of the drug. The popular demand for experts on cocaine far exceeds the supply. Public information often comes from anointed authorities who may have little experience or perspective but are willing to make public statements. Scientists have a particularly difficult task. Their real information is restricted to their data and a critical knowledge of the literature. The media's need for authoritative rather than expert statements encourages researchers to extrapolate results. This "truth" is particularly susceptible to misinterpretation. A scientist's research may be pertinent to pharmacology and irrelevent to street drug abuse. The lurid substrate of murder, Mafia, and political revolution makes our scientific knowledge seem prosaic by comparison.

OUR KNOWLEDGE OF THE DRUG: A HISTORY

The history of scientific knowledge of cocaine indicates that its most pertinent properties have long been recognized. The uses of these properties change over time. Native to South America, cocaine is derived from the leaves of the shrub *Erythroxylon*, of which over 200 species are known. No written history precedes the Conquest in 1532 but tradition has it, and archeological finds support it, that the leaves have been masticated and sucked for mental, religious, sacramental, or nutritive sustenance for millennia. The persistence of the habit points to a constant reinforcer, and all modern evidence indicates the alkaloid, cocaine, which can be found in concentrations of up to 1.8% of leaf weight. We do not know the patterns of usage in the many pre-Inca civilizations, although the numerous representations of coca consumption indicate that it may well have been a commonplace of Indian life. Although the iconography is complex, Moche line drawings on pottery indicate that it was used in ritual and that its psychoactive properties were marked (Donnan, 1978). We know from pottery images that alkali lime, usually in the form of a paste, was invariably used in conjunction with the coca leaves.

Knowledge of coca use in pre-Inca times is based on archeology. Since hardly any of the written information about Inca use comes from Inca sources, so much of what is accepted as history must be considered speculation. Drug use is hard enough to track in modern times. The written histories are either Spanish, for example Cieza de Leon (1550), or from acculturated descendants of the Incas, such as Garcilaso de la Vega (1609, 1617). It is not unreasonable to speculate that certain applications of the herbal form have remained unchanged for thousands of years and so studies of unacculturated but modern users can give us some insight into uses of the drug. Further, Indian use is not peculiar to high altitudes; jungle tribes with ritual coca use have been described (Schultes, 1981). It was not until recently that anyone examined the simple question of whether the lime or llipta used by the Indians aids in the extraction of cocaine from the leaf (it does not) or rather, by changing the pH, increases the bioavailability of the drug (it does) (Rivier, 1981). The stimulant effect of coca, reducing fatigue and hunger and improving mood, has probably been known for thousands of years and was the presumed basis for its use by the pre-Inca and Inca civilizations.

The results of chronic and continuous use of coca have been known for centuries and were explicitly delineated for cocaine by Lewin (1924). The high dependency potential of the alkaloid was set forth in the late 19th century. Acute psychoses and paranoid states were described at the same time. Despite this, there are few if any documented modern reports of cocaine psychosis and the best psychological descriptions are from before 1930. We still do not know what dose or what plasma level accompanies psychotic phenomena, nor do we know whether this is an inevitable or idiosyncratic effect of the drug. The general pharmacology of cocaine was described by von Anrep and others (Anrep, 1880; Moreno y Maiz, 1868), and the central effects were vividly described by Freud in his review *Über Coca* (1884).

Some facts of cocaine are straightforward and easily observed without "science." It numbs mucous membranes—undoubtedly known for 1000 years. It can be used as a local anesthetic—surprisingly deduced only 100 years ago. (The speculation that ancient Peruvian trephining was done with the aid of coca is unsupported by any evidence.) The discovery of local anesthesia by Carl Koller (Liljestrand, 1967; Koller-Becker, 1962) is curious in that it was a discovery of an application, not a property, of cocaine. The same is true of the development of nerve block anesthesia by Hall and Halsted (Hall, 1884).

In both instances earlier investigators had both done the experiments and reported the results, but the connection to practice was not made. Once the practical usage was demonstrated there was an explosion of interest in legitimate medical applications of cocaine. Despite the discovery of synthetic local anesthetics, cocaine is still preferred by many physicians because of its combination of vasoconstrictive and local anesthetic effects. Cocaine is no longer used in ophthalmic surgery since it can produce corneal lesions, but it is still unsurpassed as a topical anesthetic prior to intubations.

Topical use leads to appreciable plasma levels (Van Dyke et al., 1976). Whatever central stimulation is produced under these conditions is not usually viewed as undesirable. There are occasional reports of toxic psychoses and even rare reports of death from topical anesthesia with cocaine alone.

As befits a panacea, many other medical uses have been proposed over the years. As a vasoconstrictor and sympathomimetic bronchodilator, it was used for asthma. There are isolated reports of generalized analgesia with cocaine (Harrison, 1911) and it has been suggested as a treatment for arthritis.

The central nervous system stimulant properties of cocaine were exploited medically in a more naive era. Although many suggestions have been made to encourage its use for the purpose, the antidepressant properties of the drug are limited by its short duration of action and questionable efficacy (Post 1974a,b). Further research in this area would be desirable since the original trials were of limited duration and scope. The possible uses of cocaine in increasing performance, both physical and mental, fall beyond the realm of therapeutic medicine.

Examination of a standard textbook of pharmacology from 1922 (Sollman, 1922) shows that the cardiovascular, respiratory, thermoregulatory, and mydriatic properties were well known. The central stimulant effects and abuse liability are described, and of course the local anesthetic actions of the drug are discussed at length. The convulsive toxicity of the drug is known and the similarity to caffeine is noted. The central action is described as following a path from elation and vigor to delusions and mania and a depression following withdrawal is described. A modern textbook (Ritchie & Green, in Goodman & Gilman, 1980) has much more to say about the mechanism of local anesthesia and adds significantly to the information about absorption, plasma levels, fate, and excretion.

The disastrous effects of heavy usage were described by Lewin and his contemporaries. Our knowledge of the phenomenology of human abuse and its consequences has not been markedly increased since that time. Beyond reports of quantifiable reinforcement in animals, very little else has been added to our knowledge of cocaine abuse in the intervening 60 years. Modern abusers have not discovered something new; they are simply buying a well-advertised commodity whose dangers have been forgotten.

Modern technical methods have been necessary to define cocaine chemically. Gaedecke in 1855 extracted coca leaves and prepared a crystalline substance with an oily residue. He called the chemical erythroxyline. Dr. Albert Nieman, an assistant to Professor V. Wohler, the "father of synthetic organic chemistry," extracted and purified a crystalline compound from coca leaves and named it cocaine in 1862. A structure was proposed in 1898 and the total synthesis was confirmed by Wilstätter et al. (1923). However, it was not until 1955 that the full stereochemical structure of cocaine was determined by Hardegger and Ott (1955).

The most important developments in our recent knowledge of the pharmacology of cocaine were techniques that allowed determinations of nanogram quantities in blood (Jatlow & Bailey, 1975; Hawks et al., 1974) and analysis of metabolites in urine (Fish & Wilson, 1969; Rubenstein et al., 1972; Bastos et al., 1974). The realization by Jatlow and his colleagues (1976) that pseudocholinesterases in the blood broke down cocaine was an equally critical discovery.

Measurement of plasma cocaine after various routes of ingestion gave additional clues about the intensity and time course of action of drug effect. Plasma levels and effects were correlated after intravenous (Javaid et al., 1978), intranasal and oral (Van Dyke et al., 1978), and smoking (Paly et al., 1980, 1982) routes of administration. Plasma levels of cocaine in coca chewers were measured by modern techniques (Holmstedt et al., 1979) and in Peruvian natives while chewing coca leaves with and without lime (Paly et al., 1980).

The most notable property of cocaine, its intense reinforcing property, has been the source of much controversy. This property was known to the early researchers on cocaine and cautions were expressed clearly in the late 19th century (Erlenmeyer, 1885, 1886). A convincing neurochemical explanation for this reinforcement eludes us. Cocaine was used widely in the study of the peripheral sympathetic nervous system because of its action in blocking the reuptake of amines. It is still fashionable to attribute its stimulant and reinforcement properties to this action. Other reuptake blockers are not euphoriants; therefore this explanation cannot be sufficient. It is, however, the most convenient and scientific-sounding description and so has been adopted by the media.

Although a great deal is known about aminergic and endorphinergic systems, and we have reasonable hypotheses about drug-induced euphoria, we do not know either the locus or mechanism or action of any of the euphorigens. This is an important area to explore, both for its drug abuse and psychiatric implications. Whether or not cocaine has unique properties in the laboratory, it does have a unique reputation that our science has so far been inadequate to explain.

HISTORY OF OPINION

The history of opinions about cocaine is a history of perceived benefit or dangerousness to individuals and to society. The positive aspects of stimulant euphoriants, of which cocaine is an exemplar, have been attacked on religious or moral grounds because of a general societal disapproval of "drugs" not included in the society's traditions. The natural source of the drug, on the other hand, encourages its advocates to propose it as akin to food and, by implication, safe. Cocaine was introduced into Europe around the same time as tobacco, coffee, tea, and chocolate. Braudel (1981) describes parallel patterns of reaction to these natural sources of psychoactive alkaloid. The idea of panaceas, multiple medical uses, condemnations, and finally integration into acceptable use patterns is the same. Cocaine, however, is the only one of these substances where use of the chemically purified alkaloid has become a problem in the modern world. Coffee and tea containing caffeine, also a CNS stimulant, have not been identified in modern times as significant drugs of abuse despite caffeine's superficial pharmacological similarity to cocaine. Modern attitudes toward tobacco have been changing despite its significant economic base. The confirmation of the health consequences of this other American leaf has diminished its glamorous image in the public mind. Efforts to document the health consequences of cocaine use may well result in a re-realization of the dangers of chronic intensive use of stimulants.

The two images of cocaine in history appear to be antithetical. Positively, it is a beneficial stimulant with a wide range of therapeutic uses, safe, nonaddicting, a natural remedy used by the elite. Negatively, it is a psychosis-producing, addicting, dangerous "narcotic," a hard drug involved with and leading to crime, used by degenerates.

Let it be said that some reasonable evidence can be adduced to support every one of these characteristics. Over time the position of society has varied. The Inca society had a most positive image of the virtue of coca. The initial Spanish image was negative but when the uses of the drug became apparent their attitude changed. For the most part, the drug was positively viewed in the 17th century; there is a curious hiatus in the 18th century; the late 19th century was the heyday of the positive viewpoint. The early 20th century moved negative. In the 1920s newspapers were again emphasizing the romance. There was relative disinterest from the mid 1930s to the mid 1960s. Once again a positive viewpoint emerged. This view, fueled by the media, increased until the early 1980s. We are now on the verge of a new downswing. This opinion shift—a repetition of history—is not just the result of political climate, it is also the result of the consequences of widespread use, itself a consequence of the drug as a successful commodity.

The turning point in modern opinion was probably the coincidence of a comedian's serious injury and a comic's death. Suddenly cocaine was no longer either fun or funny. *Time* (1983) now headlined "Fighting Cocaine's Grip." *US News and World Report* showed a woman snorting through a glass tube from a small pile of powder and headed its cover "How Drugs Sap the Nation's Strength" (McBee, 1983). The *New York Times* reported realistically on several drugs, including both cocaine and alcohol (Schmeck, 1983; Gross, 1983). The reputation of cocaine as a safe and harmless material is once again being revised.

How does this come about? It is possible that the euphoria about euphoriants leads to indiscriminate use. A larger population at risk results in more cases of toxicity and wider exposure to drug dependency. The information sources that fed the expansion now turn to condemnation. The alkaloid cannot meet the expectations of wondrous properties without risk. It becomes a major illegal trade item and is associated with organized crime. A period of revulsion follows and once again the drug is viewed as a dangerous villain. Our pattern of learning about the drug is discontinuous but cumulative. The history of opinion is determined by rediscovery of previously reported information. With cocaine there is little news, only rediscoveries.

CURRENT ISSUES

The current issues about cocaine are social, economic, and pharmacological. Millions of people have tried it, billions of dollars are spent on it, and an explanation of its central action escapes us. Cocaine is used by a wide range of individuals. Often we find that the most accomplished are most pervasively destroyed by the drug. The damage to the nation's productive individuals is a major source of concern. The social acceptability and desirability of the substance lead to a wider exposure of individuals, a certain number of whom will become involved with compulsive use. Neither physicians nor users can predict who will become an intensive user. The high cost has limited the damage but falling prices pose a new threat. As stated earlier, the form of the drug and the route of administration are also critical determinants of the use patterns and so the effects on society.

There has been a recent change in use patterns with the introduction of free-base smoking (Byck, 1980; Siegel, 1982). We do not know a great deal about cocaine smoking, but we do know enough to classify it as a highly dangerous activity. The health dangers of this practice need better documentation. We need to know a great deal more about methods of reducing or preventing cocaine use—that is both an educational and pharmacological problem. Early reports of successful cocaine-abuse treatment must still be viewed with skepticism although controlled studies are under way in various centers.

The concept of dangerousness needs to be better defined in the public consciousness. Putting aside the exaggerated fantasies that make good copy, one must recognize that individual or societal danger is related to both the properties of the drug and the population at risk. Although laboratory experiments in carefully screened subjects rarely produce adverse effects, this does not imply that the drug is safe for self-administration. The low rate of complication of cocaine anesthesia in medical practice speaks only for its safety when administered by anesthesiologists. Morphine is also "safe" under these conditions. The effects of moderate chronic use of cocaine, whether benign or malignant, are nonetheless not properly documented, and despite many efforts we still do not have a reasonable estimate of the percentage of users who get into trouble. For that matter we do not know how many users there really are.

It is unfortunate that dangerousness is often equated with the probability of causing death. By this standard many medically useful drugs are far more dangerous than cocaine. The concepts of acute and chronic phenomena in dangerousness must be made clear. Alcohol is both acutely and chronically dangerous. Cigarettes are safe acutely but dangerous chronically. Moderate amounts of cocaine can be safe or dangerous acutely, dangerous in intensive use, and either "safe" in terms of physical damage or very dangerous in terms of net effect on the individual in chronic use. Dosage, form, and route as well as the makeup of the individual user are critical variables for these and all drugs.

Long-term physical harm is also related to intensity of use and route of administration. We do not know what percentage of occasional users become intensive users. Certain routes of administration, smoking and intravenous, almost surely are higher risk activities and thus more dangerous than oral or intranasal administration. Intensive intranasal use is not, however, rare in groups with easy access to the drug.

Simplistic beliefs, based on unwarranted amplifications of correct scientific information, lead to misinterpretation of safety. Confusion over terminology, such as the use of the words "addicting" and "narcotic," must be clarified. It is immaterial whether cocaine is addicting by any of the strict medical definitions. There is ample evidence that it can be a cause of a compulsive and personally damaging pattern of use. Regardless of legal definition, it is nonsense to insist that cocaine is a narcotic. By any scientific usage it is a central stimulant and shares no actions with narcotics.

The economic impact of a multibillion dollar untaxed illegal "industry" which subverts law enforcement and reporting in the media while influencing the activities of legitimate businesses is immense. Our country cannot afford the cocaine habit.

The effect on international relations of the gigantic cocaine trade is also a cause of major concern. Although we are not innocent of exporting dangerous drugs of abuse ourselves, the economic consequence is so severe that we must devise methods to control the flow of drugs in and dollars out. It is of course tragic that the very countries involved in cocaine export are often those with the greatest governmental monetary difficulties.

It is reasonable to suggest that the public information problem is the major cocaine issue. This chapter clearly indicates that perceptions of a drug affect its usage pattern. The possibilities or acceptance that media presentations of cocaine are affected by the use of the drug by members of the media should be explored. Although completely undocumented, it is hard to believe that an "industry" of these dimensions has no influence on public perceptions.

The presentation of confirmed and believable information about cocaine or any other drug of abuse requires continued research and clear presentation of findings. It is characteristic of science that answers must always be qualified and it is characteristic of the media that the qualifications never appear in the headlines. Research into human behavior with drugs has inherent limitations. We can and have found out much about the substance itself. We need more carefully assembled, accurate information about use patterns and liabilities of drug use. Even though cocaine is a drug of abuse, we should not be frightened from telling the truth. Its use as a pharmacological tool in the study of euphoria is yet to be properly exploited. Reduction in drug usage of all kinds requires both a knowledge of and respect for the two-edged nature of the substances. This can be transmitted by responsible use of the media and responsible behavior by the media.

The histories of cocaine provide an important message. We still have unanswered scientific questions, but our ability to use the information we have is now limited by impaired transmission of information and our inability to learn from the past.

NOTES

The pattern of distortion is obvious and was noted by readers (Harris, 1982; Emery, 1982) and other news media (Woods, 1982). Television news is often taken off the wires, which are derived from reports that may have already induced bias. The further contraction of information can cause even greater distortion. Here the telecast report is compared with relevant parts of the article from which it claims to be drawn.

1. *"No more harmful . . . than . . . cigarettes or . . . alcohol."*
   "We have legalized both alcohol and tobacco which, although pleasurable to some people, are distinct hazards to both personal and public health." (No direct comparison in health effects is made with cocaine.)
2. *"A six year study of cocaine use . . . "*
   "After six years of work on the problem our group at Yale University has been able to describe the time course of the basic pharmacological effects." (There is no mention of a cocaine *use* study, rather than a study in clinical pharmacology. This particular error is common in science reporting but can, as in this case, lead to an incorrect impression of what new findings have been revealed.)
3. *"Concludes . . . the drug is relatively safe."*
   "Medically, cocaine is a relatively safe drug but in the hands of naive

people it can lead to self-destructive behavior." (Medical use, i.e., anesthesia, is relatively safe; the article clearly states the dangers of self administration.)

4. *If not taken in large amounts . . . not addictive.*
"On the other hand cocaine certainly is addicting within the broader sense of the term that has now been adopted by many pharmacologists." (The "amount" has of course nothing to do with the dependency potential since, if an addiction occurs, "large amounts" will be taken.)

REFERENCES

Aldrich, M.R., Barker, R.W. (1976) Historical aspects of cocaine use and abuse. In Mule, S.J. (ed.), *Cocaine: Chemical, Biological, Clinical, Social and Treatment Aspects.* Cleveland: CRC Press, pp. 1–11.

Andersen, K. (1983) Crashing on cocaine. *Time* 121(15):22–31.

Anrep, v., V. (1880) Uber die physiologische Wirkung des Cocain. *Pflügers Arch* 21:38–77.

Ashley, R. (1975) *Cocaine: Its History, Uses and Effects.* New York: St. Martin's Press.

Bastos, M.L., Jukofsky, D., Mule, S.J. (1974) Routine identification of cocaine metabolites in human urine. *J. Chromatogr.* 89:335–342.

Braudel, F. (tr. Sian Reynolds). (1981) *The Structures of Everyday Life, Civilization and Capitalism 15th–18th Century*, Vol. I. New York: Harper & Row, pp. 249–265.

Byck, R. (ed.) (1974) *Cocaine Papers: Sigmund Freud.* New York: Stonehill. [Paperback. New York: New American Library, 1975].

Byck, R. (1980) Cocaine: a major drug issue of the seventies. In: *Hearings 96th Congress.* Washington, D.C.: U.S. Government Printing Office, pp. 58–69 and 88–93.

Cabieses de Molina, F. (1975) The antifatigue action of cocaine and habituation to coca in Peru. In Andrews, G. and Solomon, D. (eds.), *The Coca Leaf and Cocaine Papers.* New York: Harcourt Brace Jovanovich, p. 268.

Churcher, S. (1978) Heroin versus cocaine: the drug of choice. *New York Magazine* 11(39): 54.

Cieza de Leon, Pedro. (1883) *The Second Part of the Chronicles of Peru (1550).* Markham, C.R., tr. and ed. London: Hakluyt Society.

Collins, G. (1983) U.S. social tolerance of drugs found on rise. *New York Times* 127:1 and B5 (March 21).

Demarest, M. (1981) (Cover story) Cocaine: middle class high. *Time* 118(1):56–63.

Donnan, C. (1978) *Moche Art of Peru, Pre-Columbian Symbolic Communication.* Los Angeles: Museum of Cultural History, Univ. of Cal., p. 118.

Emery, J.L. (1982) Letter to *Hartford Courant*, March 13.

Erlenmeyer, A. (1886) Über cocainsucht. *Deutsche Medizinal-Zeitung* 7: 383–384.

Erlenmeyer, A. (1885) Über die Wirkung des Cocain bei der Morphiumentziehung. *Centralbl d Nervenheilkunde* 8:289–299 (July).

Fish, F., Wilson, W.D.C. (1969) Excretion of cocaine and its metabolites in man. *J. Pharm. Pharmacol.* 21: 1355.

Freud, S. (1884) Über coca. *Centralbl f d ges Therapie* 2:289–314 (July).

Garcilaso de la Vega. Comentarios Reales de los Incas. la. parte 1609, 2a. parte 1617, Cordova. La segunda parte tambien como: *Historia General del Peru*, edicion al cuidado de Angel Rosenblar, 3 vols. Buenos Aires: Emece Editores, 1944. [Tr. by Livermore. Austin: University of Texas Press, 1966.]

Grinspoon, L., Bakalar, J.B. (1976) *Cocaine: A Drug and Its Social Evolution.* New York: Basic Books.

Gross, J. (1983) Drug addiction: the cost to sports keeps growing in 1983. *New York Times*, July 25, pp. C1 and C6.

Hall, R.J.(1884) (letter) *N.Y. Med. J.*, 15: 643 Dec. 6 [quoted in full in *Coca Erythroxylon and Its Derivatives*. Detroit & New York: Parke Davis & Co., 1885, pp. 37–39.]

Hardegger, v., E., Ott, H. (1955) Konfiguration des Cocain und Derivate der Ecogoninsäure. *Helv. Chim. Acta.* 38:312–320.

Harris, D. (1982) Dangers of cocaine use. *Newsday*, March 5.

Harris, R. (1971) *Death of a Revolutionary*. New York: Collier Books, p. 21.

Harrison, P.W. (1911) The intravenous use of cocaine: report of a case. *Bost. Med. Surg. J.* 164:151.

Hawks, R.L., Kopin, I.J., Colburn, R.W., Thoa, N.B. (1974) Norcocaine: a pharmacologically active metabolite of cocaine found in brain. *Life Sci.* 15: 2189.

Helfand, W.H. (1980) Vin Mariani. *Pharmacy in History* 22(1):11–19.

Holmstedt, B., Fredga, A.(1981) Sundry episodes in the history of coca and cocaine. *J. Ethnopharmacol.* 3:113–147.

Holmstedt, B., Lindgren, J., Rivier, L.(1979) Cocaine in the blood of coca chewers. *J. Ethnopharmacol* 1:69.

Jatlow, P.I., Bailey, D.N. (1975) Gas-chromatographic analysis for cocaine in human plasma, with use of a nitrogen detector. *Clin. Chem.* 21:1918–1921.

Jatlow, P., Barash, P.G., Van Dyke, C., Byck, R. (1976) Impaired hydrolysis of cocaine in plasma from succinylcholine sensitive individuals. *Clin. Res.* 24:255A.

Javaid, J.I., Fischman, M.W., Schuster, C.R., Dekirmenjian, H., Davis, J.M. (1978) Cocaine plasma concentration: relation to physiological and subjective effects in humans. *Science* 202: 227–228.

Koller-Becker, H. (1962) Carl Koller and cocaine. *Psychoanal. Q.* 32:309–373.

Lewin, L. (1924, 1931) *Phantastica.* Berlin: Georg Stilke, 1924; Wirth, P.H.A. (tr. from 2nd German edition). *Phantastica, Narcotic and Stimulating Drugs, Their Use and Abuse.* London: Kegan Paul, Trench, & Trubner, 1931.

Liljestrand, G. (1967) Carl Koller and the development of local anesthesia. *Acta. Physiol. Scand. [Suppl]* 299: 30.

Liljestrand, G. (1963) Local anesthetics. In Holmstedt, B. and Liljestrand, G., eds., *Readings in Pharmacology.* Oxford: *Pergamon Press*, pp. 155–168.

Martin, R.T. (1970) The role of coca in the history, religion and medicine of South American Indians. *Economic Botany*, 24: 422–438.

McBee, S. (with Peterson, S.) (1983) Special report: How drugs sap the nation's strength. *US News & World Report* 94(19):55–58.

Moreno y Maiz, T. (1868) *Recherches Chimiques et Physiologiques sur l'Erythroxylum coca du Perou et la Cocaine.* Paris: Louis Leclerc.

Mortimer, W.G. (1901) *Peru: History of coca.* New York: J.H. Vail [Repr. San Francisco: And/Or Press, 1974].

Musto, D. (1973) *The American Disease: Origins of Narcotic Control.* New Haven: Yale University Press.

New York Herald. (1913) 10 Killed, 35 hurt in race riot born of a cocaine "jag": drug crazed Negroes fire at every one in sight in Mississippi town, Sept. 29, 1913, p.1.[Quoted in G. Silver ed., *The Dope Chronicles.* San Francisco: Harper & Row, 1979, p. 55.]

New York Magazine. (1978) Cover photo. 11(39): Sept. 25.

O'Toole, T. (1982) Cocaine behavior. *Washington Post*, Feb. 25, pp. 1–2.

Paly, D., Jatlow, P., Van Dyke, C., Cabieses, F., Byck, R. (1980) Plasma levels of cocaine in native peruvian coca chewers. In Jeri, F.R., ed., *Cocaine 1980.* Lima: Pacific Press, pp. 86–89.

Paly, D., Van Dyke, C., Jatlow, P., Barash, P., Byck, R. (1980) Cocaine: plasma levels after cocaine paste smoking. In Jeri, F.R., ed., *Cocaine 1980.* Lima: Pacific Press, pp. 106–110.

Paly, D., Jatlow, P., Van Dyke, C., Jeri, F.R., Byck, R. (1982) Cocaine paste smoking: plasma levels and effects. *Life Sci* 30: 731–738.

Petersen, R.C. (1977) History of cocaine. In Petersen, R.C. and Stillman, R.C., eds., *Cocaine: 1977.* NIDA Research Monograph #13. Rockville, Md.: DHEW, pp. 17–34.

Post, R.M., Gillin, J.C., Wyatt, R.J., Goodwin, F.K. (1974a) The effect of orally administered cocaine on sleep of depressed patients. *Psychopharmacol.* 37:59–66.

Post, R.M., Kotin, J., Goodwin, F.K.(1974b) The effects of cocaine on depressed patients. *Am. J. Psychiatry* 131:511–517.

Ritchie, J.M., Greene, N.M. (1980) Local anesthetics. In Gilman, A.G., Goodman, L.S., and Gilman, A., eds., *The Pharmacological Basis of Therapeutics*, 6th edition. New York: Macmillan, pp. 300–320.

Rivier, L. (1981) Analysis of alkaloids in leaves of cultivated *Erythroxylum* and characterization of alkaline substances used during coca chewing. *J. Ethnopharmacol.* 3:313–335.

Rubenstein, K.E., Schneider, R.S., Vilman, E.F. (1972) "Homogeneous" enzyme immunoassay. A new immunochemical technique. *Biochem. Biophys. Res. Commun.* 47:846.

Schmeck, H.J. (1983) Drug abuse in America. *New York Times*, March 22, pp. C1 and C10.

Schultes, R.E. (1981) Coca in the northwest Amazon. *J. Ethnopharmacol.* 3:173–194.

Siegel, R.K. (1982) Cocaine smoking. *J. Psychoactive Drugs* 14(4):271–359.

Sollman, T. (1922) *A Manual of pharmacology*, 2nd edition. Philadelphia & London: W.B. Saunders.

Time. (1983) Cover photo. 121(15):April 11.

Time. (1981) Cover photo. 118(1):July 6.

US News & World Report. (1983) Cover photo. 94(19): May 16.

Van Dyke, C., Barash, P.G., Jatlow, P., Byck, R. (1976) Cocaine plasma concentrations after intranasal application in man. *Science* 191: 859–861.

Van Dyke, C., Byck, R. (1982) Cocaine. *Sci Am* 246:128–141.

Van Dyke, C., Jatlow, P., Ungerer, J., Barash, P.G., Byck, R. (1978) Oral cocaine: plasma concentrations and central effects. *Science* 200:211–213.

Willstätter, R., Wolfes, O., Mader, H. (1923) Syntheses des Natürlichen Cocaines. *Justus Liebigs Annalen d Chemie* 434:111.

Woods, M. (1982) Popular beliefs about cocaine use are very dangerous. *Toledo Blade*, March 17.

ACKNOWLEDGMENT

Carol Sussman of NIDA supplied many newspaper and television references. Susan Wheeler, Edward Huberman, Frank Gawin, and Mary Ahern all provided valuable assistance.

2 | Reinforcing and Discriminative Stimulus Effects of Cocaine: Analysis of Pharmacological Mechanisms

JAMES H. WOODS, GAIL D. WINGER,
and CHARLES P. FRANCE

ANIMAL MODELS of various human illnesses have proven over the years to be extremely helpful in providing a better understanding of the causes of many diseases, their development, and possible methods of treatment. This has been no less true when the "disease" in question is not the result of an interaction between an infectious agent and the body of a human or animal host, but between a drug of abuse and the behavior of the organism. Animal models have provided a surprisingly congruent picture of the relevant effects of drugs of abuse and, in so doing, have helped determine which new drugs are likely to be abused, what pharmacological interventions may be helpful in the treatment of drug abuse, and what the potential mechanisms of action are of an abused drug. Animal models have also made it clear that more than just the pharmacology of a drug is important in determining the characteristics of its abuse. For example, both the current and historical contingencies that link or have linked the organism's behavior to delivery of the drug are very important determinants of drug-taking behavior.

The purpose of this chapter is to describe some of the human and animal research that has attempted to establish connections between the behavioral effects and the pharmacology of cocaine. Studies that demonstrate a critical interaction between current or historical contingencies and the behavioral effects of cocaine are also reviewed. The behavioral effects that will be emphasized are those mediated by the discriminative and reinforcing stimulus properties of cocaine, since these properties appear relevant to the abuse of this drug. The pharmacological actions that are currently best understood, and will therefore be stressed, are the dopamine agonist effects of cocaine and the local anesthetic properties of this drug. If the animal and human research can determine how the pharmacology of cocaine is related to its discriminative stimulus and reinforcing effects, the chances that medicinal chemists can develop effective chemotherapeutic agents for the treatment of cocaine abuse are greatly enhanced. By the same token, behavioral approaches to treatment that complement pharmacological ones might be investigated; at present, virtually no experimental effort has been devoted to these important combined objectives.

UNCONDITIONED BEHAVIORAL EFFECTS OF COCAINE

In addition to discriminative stimulus and reinforcing effects, cocaine has other behavioral effects. Because these other effects may influence results obtained in studies of the discriminative stimulus and reinforcing effects of cocaine, they will be described briefly.

Cocaine produces convulsions at large doses, and the lethal effects of cocaine are usually associated with these convulsions and the concomitant cardiovascular and respiratory dysfunction. Unconditioned and conditioned behaviors are modified by cocaine at smaller doses—those associated with most self-administration situations. For example, locomoter activity is increased by relatively small doses of cocaine; larger doses produce stereotyped behavior. The effects of cocaine on operant behavior maintained by stimuli other than cocaine depend both on the dose of cocaine that is administered and the rate of ongoing responding. Low rates of responding are increased more than high rates by intermediate doses of cocaine. Larger doses may increase low rates of responding while decreasing high rates of responding; very large doses of cocaine decrease responding regardless of the rate.

Cocaine will presumably exert unconditioned effects on behavior in any situation in which it is administered, regardless of the contingencies of cocaine delivery. In the discussions below on the discriminative stimulus and reinforcing effects of cocaine, it must be kept in mind that, even when the unconditioned effects of this drug are not of primary interest, they are probably still occurring and may influence the behavior that is being measured. Illustrations of these effects of cocaine on self-administration behavior will be given later.

NEURONAL ACTIONS OF COCAINE

The pharmacology of cocaine as it relates to its behavioral effects is complicated and as yet poorly understood. Cocaine has many actions on nervous tissue, but it is not known in detail how these actions are related to the effects of cocaine on behavior. It is now well established that cocaine blocks the reuptake of released monoamines including norepinephrine, dopamine, and serotonin. This blockade results in an accumulation of biogenic amines in the synaptic cleft, and consequently the effects of these neurotransmitters are augmented. It has been suggested that cocaine's capacity to block the reuptake of catecholamines may account for its psychomotor stimulant effects. There is a significant body of evidence that fails to support the simplest form of this hypothesis, since tricyclic antidepressants are also very effective blockers of catecholamine reuptake, yet they share very few behavioral effects with cocaine. They do not, for example, increase locomotor activity, produce convulsions, or act as positive reinforcers in animals.

The behavioral effects of amphetamine are very much like those of cocaine. These two drugs have similar unconditioned effects on behavior, maintain drug-taking behavior, have discriminative stimulus properties in common, and have effects that are, with a few interesting exceptions, antagonized by the same drugs. The primary behavioral difference between amphetamine and cocaine appears to be that cocaine has a markedly shorter duration of action, yet the neuropharmacological actions of the two compounds appear to be different. While amphetamine causes a release of catecholamines and, under some circumstances, may act directly on neurotransmitter receptors, cocaine has not been shown to exert either of these actions. Presumably there is a common denominator in the pharmacology of these two drugs that will eventually be uncovered as we understand more about how the pharmacological actions of each drug are related to its behavioral effects.

Cocaine has a membrane stabilizing action that produces local anesthesia. This effect of cocaine, however, is not shared by other psychomotor stimulants. Local anesthetics in general do not increase locomotor activity nor do they produce strong rate-dependent actions. Some local anesthetics, however, function as positive reinforcers, and it remains to be determined whether cocaine's reinforcing effects are related to its local anesthetic actions.

DISCRIMINATIVE STIMULUS EFFECTS OF COCAINE

Upon administration of appropriate doses of cocaine, humans report feelings of increased well-being, euphoria, increased energy, and decreased fatigue (e.g., Fischman & Schuster, 1982). Although animals cannot as readily indicate these types of affective changes produced by stimulant administration, they nevertheless can be trained to detect and report the presence or absence of a particular drug. In a typical discrimination experiment animals are trained to make one of two responses following administration of a stimulant drug, and the other response following the administration of a vehicle solution (e.g., saline). Only responding on the correct (i.e., injection-appropriate) response alternative produces reinforcement. A variety of infrahuman species can be trained to respond differentially in the presence or absence of drug, indicating that the drug can serve as a discriminative stimulus. Once the discrimination is acquired, compounds other than the training drug are administered and the degree to which they produce responding on the drug-associated response alternative is used as an index of similarity of interoceptive stimulus effects. Thus, subjects make the drug-associated response when compounds are administered that have stimulus properties in common with the training drug, while other compounds produce responding on the non-drug response alternative. This procedure allows for a quantitative evaluation of the discriminative stimulus properties of a wide variety of drugs.

The stimulant most commonly used as a discriminative stimulus has been amphetamine. Its stimulus effects appear to be centrally mediated and may be pharmacologically selective (Ho & McKenna, 1978; Huang & Ho, 1974c). Nevertheless, cocaine produces amphetamine-appropriate responding in virtually all situations in which it has been evaluated. More recently, cocaine itself has been used to establish a discrimination. In animals trained to discriminate one psychomotor stimulant from vehicle, there is a symmetrical cross-generalization between cocaine, amphetamine, and similar psychomotor stimulants such as methylphenidate (Colpaert et al., 1979; D'Mello & Stolerman, 1977; McKenna & Ho, 1980; Silverman & Ho, 1977). Despite a general lack of understanding of the mechanism of action by which cocaine exerts discriminative stimulus effects, these effects of cocaine and psychomotor stimulants appear to be pharmacologically selective since cocaine, amphetamine, and methylphenidate reliably substitute for each other, while drugs from other pharmacological classes (with a few notable exceptions, such as propranolol) do not reliably substitute for cocaine (Tables 2.1 and 2.2).

The subjective effects of cocaine and amphetamine administered intravenously (i.v.) in human subjects are indistinguishable (Fischman et al., 1976). Other drugs which produce subjective effects in humans that are similar to those of amphetamine and cocaine are dextroamphetamine, methamphetamine, phenmetrazine, methylphenidate, and diethylpropion (Griffith et al., 1972; Jasinski et al., 1974; Martin et al., 1971).

Drug discrimination studies in animals have generally supported the notion that cocaine acts, in part, through dopaminergic systems (e.g., Schechter & Cook, 1975). Apomorphine, a drug that acts directly on central dopamine receptors, has been shown to produce cocaine-appropriate responding in many situations (Colpaert & Janssen, 1982; McKenna & Ho, 1980), while other direct dopamine agonists such as piribedil and bromocryptine do not reliably substitute for cocaine (Colpaert et al., 1979). Some compounds that are not psychomotor stimulants, but are known to increase availability of dopamine centrally (e.g., phencyclidine), do produce considerable cocaine-appropriate responding in some situations (e.g., Colpaert et al., 1979). Monoamine oxidase (MAO) inhibitors also increase functional availability of endogenous dopamine, and those which are believed to inhibit selectively type B MAO (e.g., deprenyl) have been shown to substitute for cocaine as discriminative stimuli (Colpaert et al., 1979, 1980). Thus, the relationship between dopamine receptor stimulation and the discriminative stimulus effects of cocaine remains unclear.

Because cocaine has potent local anesthetic effects, possible similarities between the discriminative stimulus effects of cocaine and other local anesthetics have been evaluated in several species, including humans. Subcutaneously administered lidocaine does not

Table 2.1 Compounds That Substitute For Cocaine as Discriminative Stimuli

Species	Cocaine Training Dose (mg/kg;route)	Test Compound (mg/kg;route)	Maximum Effect (%)	Reference
Rat	10.0; s.c.	d-amphetamine (0.31; s.c.)	100	Colpaert et al., 1979
	10.0; s.c.	Apomorphine (0.31; s.c.)	100	Colpaert et al., 1976
	10.0; s.c.	Methylphenidate (1.25; s.c.)	100	Colpaert et al., 1979
	10.0; s.c.	Nomifensine (0.63; s.c.)	100	Colpaert et al., 1979
	10.0; i.p.	Norcocaine (10.0; i.p.)	95	McKenna et al., 1979
	5.0; i.p.	N-allylnorcocaine (20.0; i.p.)	100	Bedford et al., 1981
	5.0; s.c.	Pargyline (40.0; s.c.)	80	Colpaert et al., 1980
	5.0; s.c.	Pheniprazine (10.0; s.c.)	100	Colpaert et al., 1980
Pigeon	2.0; i.m.	d-amphetamine (2.0; i.m.)	100	de la Garza & Johanson, 1985
	2.0; i.m.	l-cathinone (2.0; i.m.)	100	de la Garza & Johanson, 1985
	5.6; i.m.	norcocaine (3.0; i.m.)	100	Jarbe, 1981
	5.6; i.m.	WIN 35,428 (3.0; i.m.)	100	Jarbe, 1981
	5.6; i.m.	WIN 35,065-2 (5.6; i.m.)	100	Jarbe, 1981
Monkey	0.25; i.m.	d-amphetamine (0.25; i.m.)	90	de la Garza & Johanson, 1983
	0.25; i.m.	l-cathinone (0.25; i.m.)	90	de la Garza & Johanson, 1983
	0.25; i.m.	Procaine (8.0; i.m.)	90	de la Garza & Johanson, 1983

*In two of three monkeys.

26

Table 2.2 Compounds That Fail To Substitute For Cocaine as Discriminative Stimuli

Species	Cocaine Training Dose (mg/kg; route)	Test Compound (mg/kg; route)	Maximum Effect (%)	Reference
Rat	10.0; i.p.	Benzoylecgonine (20.0; i.p.)	20	McKenna et al., 1979
	10.0; i.p.	Benzoylnorecgonine (20.0; i.p.)	18	McKenna et al., 1979
	10.0; i.p.	Cocaine methiodide (20.0; i.p.)	34	McKenna & Ho, 1980
	10.0; s.c.	Clorgyline (40.0; s.c.)	20	Colpaert et al., 1979
	10.0; i.p.	Ecgonine (20.0; i.p.)	15	McKenna et al., 1979
	10.0; i.p.	Fenfluramine (5.0; i.p.)	17	McKenna & Ho, 1980
	10.0; s.c.	Lidocaine (10.0; s.c.)	0	Colpaert et al., 1979
	10.0; s.c.	Procaine (10.0; s.c.)	0	Colpaert et al, 1979
	10.0; i.p.	Procaine (40.0; i.p.)	55	McKenna & Ho, 1980
	10.0; i.p.	Strychnine (1.0; i.p.)	33	McKenna & Ho, 1980
Pigeon	5.6; i.m.	Hydroxyamphetamine (3.8; i.m.)	3	Jarbe, 1981
	2.0; i.m.	Lidocaine (16.0; i.m.)	30	de la Garza & Johanson, 1985
	5.6; i.m.	LSD (0.1; i.m.)	16	Jarbe, 1981
	5.6; i.m.	Morphine (5.6; i.m.)	17	Jarbe, 1981
	2.0; i.m.	Nicotine (4.0; i.m.)	70	de la Garza & Johanson, 1985
	2.0; i.m.	Oxazepam (4.0; i.m.)	0	de la Garza & Johanson, 1985
	2.0; i.m.	Pentobarbital (8.0; i.m.)	30	de la Garza & Johanson, 1985
	5.6; i.m.	Procaine (30.0; i.m.)	40	Jarbe, 1981
Monkey	0.1; i.v.	Chlorpromazine (0.4; i.v.)	20	Ando & Yanagita, 1978
	0.1; i.v.	Ethyl alcohol (400.0; i.v.)	0	Ando & Yanagita, 1978
	0.25; i.m.	Pentobarbital (8.0; i.m.)	20	de la Garza & Johanson, 1983

27

substitute for cocaine in rats (Colpaert et al., 1979) or pigeons (de la Garza & Johanson, 1985) trained to discriminate cocaine from vehicle, whereas procaine substitutes for cocaine in some experimental situations (e.g., de la Garza & Johanson, 1983), but not all (e.g., Colpaert et al., 1979; de la Garza & Johanson, 1985; Jarbe, 1981; McKenna & Ho, 1980). Human subjects with a history of cocaine self-administration are unable to distinguish the intranasal administration of the local anesthetic lidocaine from cocaine (Van Dyke et al., 1978). It is likely, however, that the route of administration as well as the extensive drug history of the subject are critical to the results obtained with lidocaine in humans. In more recent studies, the subjective effects of lidocaine administered i.v. are reported to be unlike cocaine, and i.v. procaine is similar although not identical to cocaine (Fischman et al., 1983a,b).

The discriminative stimulus effects of cocaine and other psychomotor stimulants are probably mediated in the CNS (McKenna & Ho, 1980; Silverman & Ho, 1977). Quaternary cocaine does not substitute for cocaine in rats (Ho & McKenna, 1978) and para-hydroxyamphetamine fails to substitute for cocaine in pigeons trained to discriminate cocaine from saline (Jarbe, 1981). Furthermore, the potency of stimulants as discriminative stimuli is increased markedly if they are administered directly into the CNS (e.g., Richards et al., 1973).

Amphetamine and cocaine are potent appetite suppressants, but the discriminative stimulus effects of these agents are not attributable simply to their anorectic effects. Fenfluramine, for example, is a potent anorectic, but fails to substitute for amphetimine in rats (Schechter & Rosecrans, 1972), and neither fenfluramine nor chlorphentermine produce amphetamine-like subjective effects in humans (Griffith, 1977; Martin et al., 1971).

The discriminative stimulus properties of cocaine and amphetimine appear not to be dependent on their capacity to increase motor activity. Iproniazid and beta-phenethylamine fail to increase locomotor activity but do substitute for amphetamine (Huang & Ho, 1974c), and local anesthetics that substitute for cocaine under some experimental conditions do not increase locomotor activity. Finally, drugs that produce gross CNS stimulation in the form of convulsions do not substitute for cocaine or amphetamine. Whereas nikethamide, strychnine, and picrotoxin cause CNS stimulation and convulsions, they do not share discriminative stimulus effects with psychomotor stimulants (Huang & Ho, 1974b). Collectively, these data on the discriminative stimulus effects of cocaine suggest considerable pharmacologic selectivity, but strong conclusions regarding the relation of cocaine to dopamine neurotransmission or local anesthetic action appear unwarranted.

DRUGS THAT MODIFY THE DISCRIMINATIVE STIMULUS EFFECTS OF COCAINE

Studies on the ability of various drugs to attenuate the discriminative stimulus effects of cocaine and other psychomotor stimulants have produced results that are in general agreement. Compounds that reduce the availability of central dopamine reliably antagonize the discriminative stimulus effects of psychomotor stimulants, while compounds that affect adrenergic, cholinergic, or serotonergic neurotransmission do not reliably affect the discriminative stimulus properties of psychomotor stimulants (Colpaert et al., 1978; Jarbe, 1978; McKenna & Ho, 1980). Although dopamine antagonists have been shown to attenuate the discriminative stimulus effects of both amphetamine and cocaine, in general larger doses of these agents are required to block the effects of cocaine and, as shown in Table 2.3, the discriminative stimulus effects of cocaine often are only partially antagonized.

The results displayed in Figure 2.1 are from experiments (Colpaert et al., 1978) in which rats are trained to discriminate between 10.0 mg/kg cocaine or 1.25 mg/kg d-amphetamine and vehicle. When each of these training drugs is administered in combination with the dopamine antagonist, haloperidol, the discriminative stimulus effects of each are attenuated, although haloperidol fails to attenuate completely the effects of cocaine up to doses that suppress responding markedly. At a dose of 0.31 mg/kg haloperidol, only 20% of the rats trained to discriminate amphetamine select the amphetamine lever, whereas more than half of the rats trained to discriminate cocaine select the cocaine lever. Interpretation of this as well as other examples of antagonism of cocaine by haloperidol are confounded by the fact that antagonism can be observed only with drug doses that suppress behavior markedly. This suppression may be due to the antagonism by haloperidol and other dopamine antagonists of endogenous dopamine systems, and

Table 2.3 Compounds That Antagonize Cocaine's Discriminative Stimulus Effects in Rats

Cocaine Test Dose (mg/kg; route)	Antagonist (mg/kg; route)	Maximum Decrease (%)	Reference
4.0 i.p.	Chorpromazine (8.0; i.p.)	60	Jarbe, 1978
10.0 s.c.	Haloperidol (0.31; s.c.)	50	Colpaert et al., 1978
10.0 i.p.	Haloperidol (0.5; i.p.)	52	McKenna & Ho, 1980
10.0 i.p.	Haloperidol (1.0; i.p.)	30	Cunningham & Appel, 1982
4.0 i.p.	Haloperidol (0.8; i.p.)	70	Jarbe, 1978
10.0 s.c.	Pimozide (2.5; s.c.)	NR	Colpaert et al., 1978
10.0 i.p.	Pimozide (1.0; i.p.)	40	McKenna et al.,1979
4.0 i.p.	Pimozide (1.0; i.p.)	60	Jarbe, 1978
5.0 i.p.	Pimozide (1.0; i.p.)	40	Ho & McKenna, 1978
10.0 i.p.	Reserpine (NR)	35	McKenna & Ho, 1980
10.0 i.p.	Reserpine (2.5; i.p.)	37	McKenna et al., 1979
10.0 s.c.	Spiperone (0.31; s.c.)	NR	Colpaert et al, 1978

NR = not reported

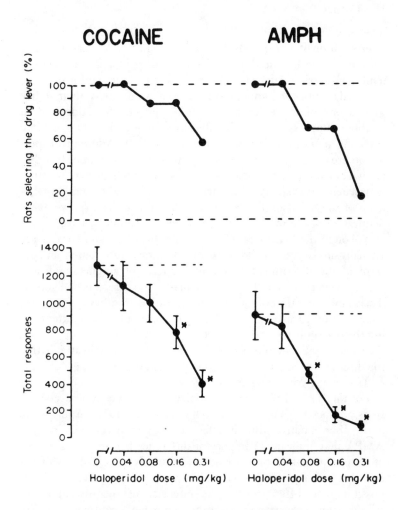

FIGURE 2.1. Antagonism of the discriminative stimulus effects of cocaine and amphetamine by haloperidol in rats trained to discriminate 10.0 mg/kg cocaine (left panels) or 1.25 mg/kg *d*-amphetamine (right panels) from saline. Abscissae: dose of haloperidol in mg/kg. Ordinates: upper panels, percentage of rats selecting the drug-appropriate key; lower panels, mean number of responses emitted during 15 minute sessions ±1 S.E.M. Haloperidol was administered 60 minutes prior to testing, cocaine or amphetamine was administered 30 minutes prior to testing. (Modified from Colpaert et al., 1978)

may be unavoidable with these compounds. It nevertheless makes interpretation of data such as those shown in Figure 2.1 very difficult, since they may be due to factors other than or in addition to attenuation of discriminative stimulus actions of cocaine. Unfortunately, a limited number of compounds have been evaluated for their ability to antagonize the discriminative stimulus effects of cocaine, and all of those suppress behavior at the doses required to demonstrate antagonism of discriminative stimulus properties. Additional experiments are needed to evaluate possible antagonism of cocaine by other known dopamine antagonists as well as compounds that act on other neurochemical systems. This lack of clear pharmacological antagonism of the behavioral effects of cocaine has, to date, prevented a delineation of the mechanism(s) of action of cocaine *in vivo*.

Although the behavioral effects of amphetamine and cocaine are virtually indistinguishable in many situations, differential antagonism of the discriminative stimulus effects of amphetamine and cocaine suggests that these drugs may not share mechanisms as discriminative stimuli. The catecholamine synthesis inhibitor, alpha-methyl-para-tyrosine (AMPT) is more effective in attentuating the discriminative stimulus effects of amphetamine; conversely, the catecholamine depleter reserpine is more effective in attenuating the discriminative effects of cocaine (Ho & Huang, 1975; McKenna & Ho, 1980; McKenna et al., 1979; Schechter & Cook, 1975). Interestingly, AMPT does antagonize the stereotypy and convulsions produced by cocaine (Wallach & Gershon, 1972). Antagonism of the discriminative stimulus effects of cocaine by reserpine but not AMPT may indicate an important difference between cocaine and other psychomotor stimulants. Unfortunately, single doses of antagonists and agonists are typically evaluated and, therefore, it is possible that differences in the intensity of the discriminative stimulus among procedures and training drugs might contribute to differences in antagonism.

While amphetamine and cocaine may have a similar or identical final common pathway through activation of central dopamine receptors, the mechanisms of this activation appear to be different. The lack of reliable substitution for cocaine by other dopamine agonists and the lack of complete antagonism of cocaine by established dopamine antagonists strongly suggest that direct activation of dopamine systems is not the only, and perhaps not the most important, action of cocaine as a discriminative stimulus. Indeed, the interoceptive stimulus produced by any drug is likely a combination of several or many independent biological effects, and may not be attributable to actions on any single neurochemical system. While stimulation of dopamine systems might be an essential action in the discriminative stimulus effects of cocaine and amphetamine, the data accumulated to date suggest that cocaine and amphetamine exert some effects that are not shared by other dopamine agonists. Thus, it is nondopaminergic actions that distinguish the discriminative stimulus effects of cocaine and amphetamine from other compounds that act, in part, on dopamine systems. If multiple mechanisms of action are important in the behavioral actions of cocaine, it is fully consistent that stimulation of any one system may be insufficient to produce discriminative stimulus effects similar to those of cocaine, and antagonism of only one system may result in only partial attenuation of a stimulus effect. It is clear that studies of the discriminative effects of cocaine and their modification by various pharmacological interventions should be accompanied by studies of as many other effects of cocaine as possible. Complete dose-effect curves, evaluation of potential antagonists in each of these systems, and comparisons of other psychomotor stimulants to cocaine are all important steps in furthering our understanding of how cocaine works and how its effects can best be prevented or reversed.

REINFORCING EFFECT OF COCAINE

That the intravenous administration of cocaine could maintain operant behavior in primates was first demonstrated by Deneau, Yanagita, and Seevers (1969). In this study, rhesus monkeys with indwelling intravenous catheters have continuous access to either 0.25 or 0.5 mg/kg/injection cocaine, contingent on a lever press response. As shown in Figure 2.2, this monkey (and others) quickly acquires the response and self-administers large amounts of cocaine. The pattern of self-administration is quite erratic; the monkey self-administers cocaine to the point of exhaustion, reduces its drug intake, and then resumes high rates of responding. The unconditioned effects of cocaine are evident in these animals in the form of restlessness, choreiform movements, stereotyped behavior, decreased food intake, and occasional convulsions.

Aigner and Balster (1978) report that monkeys given the opportunity to respond for either food or intravenous cocaine respond almost exclusively for cocaine over an eight-day period. Marked weight loss and behavioral toxicity develop over this period.

The toxicity of self-administered cocaine can be reduced considerably by restricting access to the drug. This serves not only to preserve the animals' health, but also to permit an evaluation of the reinforcing effects of the drug with less interference by unconditioned effects. The most common procedure for limiting access to cocaine is to restrict the time available for cocaine self-administration, and in some cases to limit as well the amount of drug that can be self-administered during access periods. Under conditions in which rhesus monkeys are given a 130-minute period, twice a day for cocaine self-administration under an FR 30 TO 10 schedule (30 responses per reinforcement; 10 min timeout after each injection), stable rates of cocaine self-administration occur and increasing the dose of cocaine from 0.03 to 0.32 mg/kg/injection leads to increased rates of responding (Fig. 2.3). At a dose larger than 0.32 mg/kg/injection, the dose-response function reverses and rates of responding decrease. This type of function in which response rates initially increase and then decrease as dose per injection increases (inverted U-shaped function) is typical with drugs that maintain self-administration behavior.

This function occurs not only with almost all self-administered drugs, but also with different schedules of reinforcement; a similar inverted U-shaped function also develops when several doses of cocaine are made available using a progressive-ratio schedule of reinforcement (Winger & Woods, 1985). A progressive-ratio schedule is one in which the number of responses necessary for drug delivery increases with each drug injection or across time. At some response requirement, animals will make less than the required number of responses per unit time, and will not obtain the injection. This response requirement is called the break point. The data shown in Figure 2.4 are obtained in an experiment where the response requirement starts at 30 and increases by 30 with each injection. A 10-minute timeout period follows each injection. Again, an inverted U-shaped function develops relating dose per injection of cocaine to the break point. Functions of this same or similar shape are also reported by Griffiths et al. (1979) in baboons using a progressive-ratio schedule in which the response requirement starts at 160 and doubles every 24 hours.

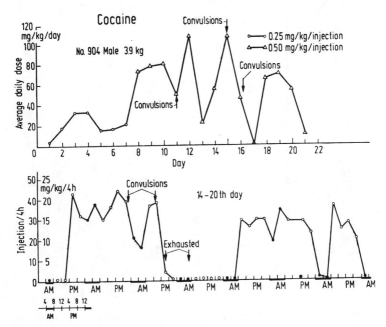

FIGURE 2.2. Pattern of cocaine self-administration in a rhesus monkey allowed continuous access to 0.25 mg/kg/injection or 0.;50 mg/kg/injection cocaine on a fixed-ratio 1 schedule of intravenous drug delivery. Ordinates: upper panel, the average daily dose of cocaine self-administration in mg/kg; lower panel, number of injections and dose (mg/kg) injected per four hours. Abscissae: time in four hour blocks. (Modified from Deneau, Yanagita & Seevers, 1969).

While the shape of the function relating dose of self-administered drug to response rate is fairly ubiquitous across drugs and schedules of reinforcement, the position of the curve along the dose axis of any particular drug can be altered markedly. One manipulation that modifies the dose-rate function for cocaine is a change in the duration of the timeout following each infusion. Downs and Woods (1974) studied self-administration of cocaine in rhesus monkeys under an FR 30 schedule with no timeout periods after the injections. The function relating dose per injection to rate of responding is shaped much like the curve shown in Figure 2.3; however, the dose that maintains peak response rates is 0.003 mg/kg/injection, 100-fold smaller than the dose that maintains

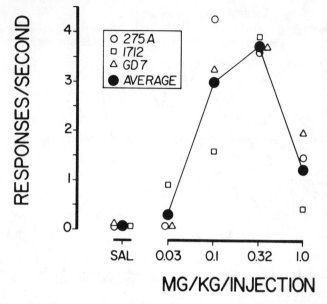

FIGURE 2.3. Intravenous self-administration of cocaine in rhesus monkeys trained to press a lever on a fixed-ratio 30 timeout 10 minutes (FR30:TO10) schedule of drug injection. A maximum of 13 injections was available during each test session. Open symbols represent data obtained from individual animals, closed symbols represent the averaged data of those three animals. Abscissae: dose of cocaine in mg/kg/injection. Ordinate: response rate expressed in responses per second. (Modified from Winger & Woods, 1985)

maximum response rates when a 10-minute timeout follows each infusion. A shift to the right in the dose of cocaine that maintained peak response rates is also shown by Griffiths et al. (1979) when the post-injection timeout is increased from 3 to 12 hours.

Procedures that induce tolerance to a drug or otherwise modify reinforcing efficacy would also change the position of the dose-rate function. In addition to altering the apparent potency of a drug, these procedures also might affect the shape of the dose-rate curve. In order to understand how the dose-rate curve could change following an alteration of the reinforcing effect of the drug, it is important to understand the apparent determinants of an inverted-U dose-effect curve.

Response rates are usually thought to reflect the strength of the

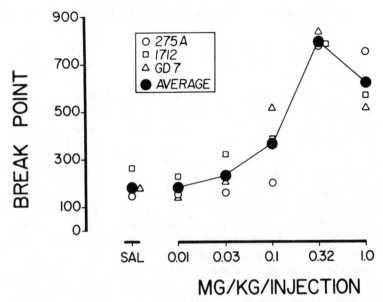

FIGURE 2.4. Breaking points for responding maintained by intravenous injections of cocaine in rhesus monkeys. The first infusion of each session was given following 30 responses. The response requirement for subsequent infusions was increased by 30 responses per infusion (e.g., 60, 90, 120 . . .). Each infusion was followed by a 10-minute timeout. The session terminated after 30 infusions or if no more than two responses occurred during a 15-minute period. The breaking point was defined as the response requirement of the last completed fixed-ratio value. Abscissae: dose of cocaine in mg/kg/injection. Ordinate: breaking point (value of last fixed-ratio). (Modified from Winger & Woods, 1985)

reinforcer used to maintain responding (Downs & Woods, 1974). Thus, as the strength of the reinforcer increases, the response rates increase as well. The cocaine dose-rate curve would, therefore, indicate that increasing the dose of cocaine increases the reinforcing strength of this drug up to some dose, after which the reinforcing efficacy of cocaine decreases. Data obtained from studies described below, however, indicate that the reinforcing efficacy of cocaine is monotonically related to dose.

Why then is there a consistent decrement in response rates at large doses of cocaine when the rate of drug self-administration is the dependent variable? The decreasing limb of drug self-administration curves is thought to be a result of the unconditioned behavioral effects of previously self-administered cocaine (Balster & Schuster, 1973; Pickens & Thompson, 1968; Wilson et al., 1971). In other words, large doses of cocaine directly suppress the rate of cocaine-reinforced responding.

A clear demonstration of the unconditioned effects of self-administered cocaine on other behavior is provided by Spealman and Kelleher (1979). In this experiment, squirrel monkeys respond on a fixed-interval (FI) schedule of reinforcement in which shock or cocaine alternately maintain schedule-controlled performance. Under one stimulus condition, responding is maintained by shock presentation; under the second stimulus condition, responding is maintained by intravenous delivery of cocaine. The rate of shock-reinforced responding is affected markedly by cocaine delivered in the alternate component of the schedule. As shown in Figure 2.5, when saline is substituted for cocaine, the rate of responding maintained by the intravenous infusions is quite low, while responding is maintained in a characteristic FI pattern during the shock presentation component of the schedule. As the dose of cocaine is increased from 10 to 300 μg/kg/injection, rates of responding maintained by shock first increases and then decreases (Fig. 2.5; Fig. 2.6, left panel). A very similar effect of cocaine on cocaine-reinforced responding is observed in two of the three monkeys (Fig. 2.6, right panel). In addition, there is a rate-dependent effect of cocaine on shock-maintained responding in that low rates are increased to a greater extent than higher rates. In this study, the unconditioned effects of self-administered cocaine are clearly demonstrated by altered rates and patterns of responding during the shock-maintained component of the schedule. Thus, unconditioned effects of self-administered cocaine clearly modify the rates and patterns of cocaine-maintained responding as well as contribute to the shape of the function that relates cocaine dose to rates of cocaine-reinforced responding.

A similar unconditioned effect of cocaine on rates of responding is observed when cocaine is administered prior to an experimental session in which monkeys are given the opportunity to self-administer cocaine. Herling et al. (1979) observe primarily decreases in rates of cocaine-maintained responding following presession, intramuscular administration of 0.3 to 5.6 mg/kg cocaine. These decreases are closely paralleled by cocaine-induced suppression of

SHOCK PRESENTATION

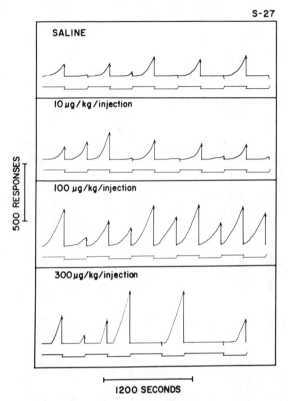

FIGURE 2.5. Responding in a squirrel monkey maintained alternately by shock presentation and intravenous cocaine injection [fixed-interval (FI) 300 seconds in both components]. The event pen was up during the shock presentation component and down during the cocaine injection component, and consecutive FI components were separated by a 1-minute timeout. Diagonal marks of the response pen indicate the presentation of shock or cocaine injection. The dose of cocaine (μg/kg/injection) is noted in each panel. (From Spealman & Kelleher, 1979)

similar rates and patterns of food-maintained responding in another group of monkeys. The effects of pretreatments with *d*-amphetamine, pentobarbital, or cocaine on the rates of responding maintained by food or cocaine appear to be determined largely by factors other than the event maintaining responding (Fig. 2.7). It thus appears that the unconditioned effects of cocaine can affect self-

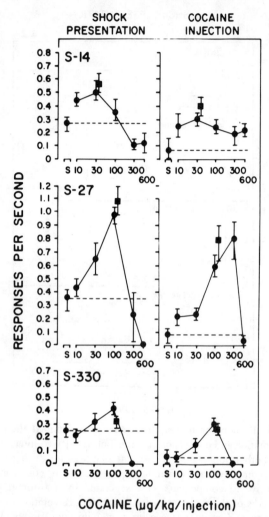

FIGURE 2.6. The effect of cocaine dose on behavior maintained alternately by intravenous cocaine injection (right panels) and electric shock presentation (left panels) in squirrel monkeys. Responding was maintained in both components by a fixed-interval (FI) 300-seconds schedule of reinforcement. Ordinates: rate of responding expressed in responses per second. Abscissae: dose of self-administered cocaine expressed in μg/kg/injection. Dashed lines represent data obtained when saline was substituted for cocaine. (From Spealman & Kelleher, 1979)

administration behavior in much the same way they affect behavior maintained by other reinforcers. Furthermore, both amphetamine and pentobarbital have similar effects on behavior maintained by either food or cocaine. If there are compounds that selectively modify the reinforcing effects of cocaine, these drugs will be identified by their differential effects on cocaine-maintained responding. This issue will be discussed further in later sections of this chapter in which the evidence for drug-induced modification of cocaine's reinforcing effects is described.

That larger doses of cocaine are more reinforcing than smaller doses has been demonstrated in studies using preference or choice behavior as the dependent variable. In studies where animals can choose between different doses of cocaine, the choice is virtually always for the larger dose. Iglauer and Woods (1974) trained rhesus monkeys in a task in which the preference for various doses of cocaine could be measured. The animals could respond on one of two levers to receive intravenous injections of cocaine. The dose of cocaine delivered following responding on one of the levers remains constant while the dose delivered following responding on the other lever varies between 0.01 and 0.8 mg/kg/injection. Preference is measured by the relative response frequency on the variable dose lever. The results shown in Figure 2.8 demonstrate clearly a dose-related preference for the larger of two doses of cocaine.

Johanson and Schuster (1975) used a choice procedure in which monkeys are given the opportunity to self-administer first one then a second dose of cocaine, each available under different stimulus conditions. The animals could subsequently choose between the doses by selecting the lever associated with one of the stimulus conditions. A dose of 0.05 mg/kg/injection is compared to 0.1, 0.2, and 0.5 mg/kg/injection, 0.1 mg/kg/injection is compared to 0.3, 0.5, and 1.5 mg/kg/injection, and 0.5 mg/kg/injection is compared to 1.0 and 1.5 mg/kg/injection. Larger doses of cocaine are preferred to smaller doses up to 0.5 mg/kg/injection. There is no apparent preference for larger doses as compared to 0.5 mg/kg/injection. At these large doses, the monkeys were extremely agitated and hyperexcitable and one animal died in convulsions. It appears, therefore, that preference for large doses of cocaine is limited only by the behavioral toxicity of the drug.

There has been only a single, formal study of cocaine self-

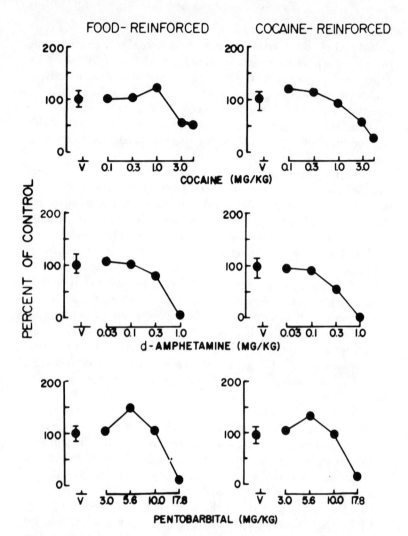

FIGURE 2.7. The effects of cocaine, *d*-amphetamine, and pentobarbital in rhesus monkeys trained to respond on a second-order fixed-interval 5-minute, fixed-ratio 10 [FI5 (FR10:S)] schedule of food delivery (left panels) or intravenous cocaine (30.0 μg/kg) injection (right panels). Abscissae: dose in mg/kg; points above V indicate the mean and range of response rates during sessions preceded by vehicle injections. Ordinates: response rate expressed as a percentage of control (i.e., vehicle pretreatment) sessions. (Modified from Herling, Downs & Woods, 1979)

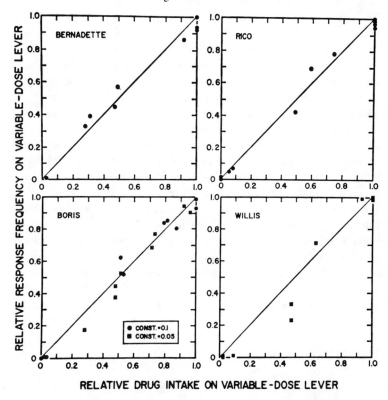

FIGURE 2.8. Dose preference for i.v. self-administered cocaine in four rhesus monkeys trained to respond on one lever for a fixed dose of cocaine (0.05 or 1.0 mg/kg/injection) and on a second lever for variable doses of cocaine (0.01 to 0.8 mg/kg/injection). Ordinates: relative response frequency on the variable-dose lever calculated as the number of responses on that lever divided by the total number of responses on both levers. Abscissae: relative drug intake on the variable-dose lever calculated as the drug intake on that lever divided by the drug intake on both levers. Drug intake was defined as the number of injections obtained on a particular lever multiplied by the available dose on that lever. The available dose on the fixed-dose lever is indicated by "CONST. = ." (From Iglauer & Woods, 1974)

administration in humans (Fischman & Schuster, 1982). The study uses a choice procedure similar to those described above in rhesus monkeys. The subjects are told that responses on a right-hand button result in intravenous cocaine infusions, while responses on a left-hand button result in intravenous infusions of saline. Forced infusions of either saline or 16 mg cocaine are then delivered every 15 minutes for one hour on the first experimental day. On the second through the tenth day, the subjects are required to press a button ten times to receive an infusion. A maximum of ten infusions could be earned in each one-hour experimental session. The subjects tend to sample both saline and cocaine during the first choice day and, thereafter, three of the four subjects choose only cocaine injections. These results clearly demonstrate the reinforcing effects of cocaine in humans under controlled experimental conditions. These investigators found that the first requested injection of cocaine produces increased heart rate and blood pressure that is accompanied by reports of a stimulant effect and a positive mood. Further requested injections result in increases in plasma levels of cocaine but no further increases in mood, stimulant effects, blood pressure, or heart rate suggesting an acute tolerance. In one subject, as shown in Figure 2.9, both the subjective reports or positive mood and stimulant effects actually decrease after the sixth injection of cocaine. These experiments illustrate a method of experimental analysis of cocaine-reinforced responding in humans that can yield new experimental information as well as extend the generality of similar studies in animals.

SELF-ADMINISTRATION OF DRUGS RELATED TO COCAINE

Local Anesthetics

Although cocaine is a psychomotor stimulant, it is also an effective local anesthetic. The discovery that the local anesthetic procaine is

---

FIGURE 2.9. Data for subject 49 on day 5, who was allowed to choose 32 mg cocaine or saline up to 10 times during a 1-hour experimental session. Arrows indicate the time at which each injection was requested. Five minutes later it was injected and cumulative cocaine intake is indicated. Plasma level, as measured after each drug choice, is shown above this. Heart rate and blood pressure were sampled every 2 minutes. Means and SEM of these measures over 30 minutes before the start of the session are indicated by small + marks to the left of the heart rate and blood pressure figures. The uppermost panels indicate a mean composite score on the POMS (positive mood, elation minus depression) and the ARCI (stimulant score, BG plus MBG plus A). (From Fischman & Schuster, 1982)

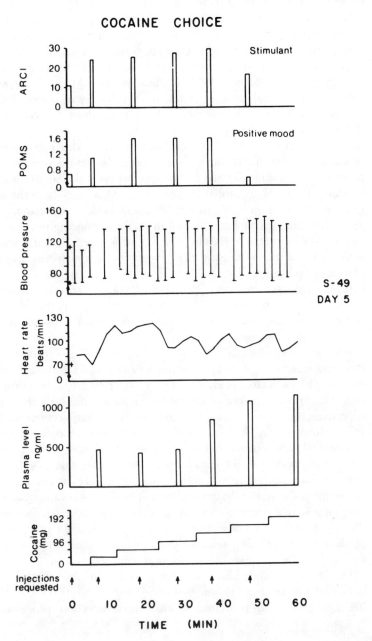

COCAINE CHOICE

S-49
DAY 5

TIME (MIN)

effective in maintaining behavior that leads to its intravenous delivery (Ford & Balster, 1977; Hammerbeck & Mitchell, 1978) raises the question of whether cocaine's reinforcing effects might be due in part to its local anesthetic action. Studies on the reinforcing effects of procaine show that it produces very little behavioral toxicity (Ford & Balster, 1977; Hammerbeck & Mitchell, 1978; Johanson, 1980) and, at some doses, maintains rates of responding that are as high or higher than those maintained by cocaine (Johanson, 1980).

Not all local anesthetics have reinforcing effects. Although chlorprocaine, a local anesthetic with a chemical structure similar to procaine, is self-administered by monkeys at rates similar to those produced by procaine, proparacaine is not taken at rates above those maintained by saline (Johanson, 1980). Lidocaine, procainamide, and diethyaminoethanol also do not maintain responding in rhesus monkeys (Woolverton & Balster, 1979). Furthermore, lidocaine has subjective effects in humans that cannot be distinguished from placebo (Fischman et al., 1983a). Thus, local anesthetics do not generally serve as reinforcers. The attributes of local anesthetics that are necessary to produce a reinforcing effect, and whether these attributes are related in any way to the reinforcing action of cocaine, are not clear at this time.

Although procaine can maintain rates of responding in excess of those maintained by cocaine, it appears to be less reinforcing than cocaine when animals can choose between the two drugs. In a drug choice experiment, a dose of 1.6 mg/kg/injection procaine is chosen only over the lowest dose of cocaine (0.05 mg/kg/injection) and saline (Johanson & Aigner, 1981). Larger doses of cocaine are consistently selected over all tested doses of procaine. The high rates of responding maintained by procaine indicate that this drug has a short duration of action and relatively insignificant rate-suppressing (unconditioned) effects. The data on cocaine choice also suggest that cocaine, since it appears to be more reinforcing that procaine but is not a more potent anesthetic than procaine, produces its reinforcing effects by mechanisms other than or in addition to those responsible for its local anesthetic actions.

De la Garza and Johanson (1982) evaluated the effects of haloperidol on behavior maintained by 0.1 mg/kg/injection cocaine, 0.4 mg/kg/injection procaine, or 1.6 mg/kg/injection procaine.

Haloperidol at a dose of 0.04 mg/kg, produces increases in cocaine-reinforced responding. This dose only decreases rates of procaine-reinforced responding, further supporting the suggestion that procaine and cocaine act via different mechanisms, at least insofar as rate-decreasing effects are concerned.

Cocaine Metabolites

The majority of administered cocaine is metabolized in the liver to the relatively inactive metabolites ecgonine and benzoylecgonine. A small amount of cocaine is metabolized to norcocaine. Norcocaine shares many effects with cocaine, including an ability to block reuptake of norepinephrine and to produce local anesthesia. Some investigators report norcocaine to have little or no ability to increase locomotor activity in rats (Bedford et al., 1980), while others find little difference in the ability of cocaine and norcocaine to affect schedule-controlled behavior in pigeons and squirrel monkeys (Spealman et al., 1979). The discriminative stimulus properties of norcocaine in rats (McKenna et al., 1979) and in pigeons (Jarbe, 1981) are similar to those of cocaine. In the rat the discriminative stimulus effects of both cocaine and norcocaine are antagonized by pimozide (McKenna et al., 1979). Norcocaine also maintains self-administration behavior in dogs under FR 1 schedules of intravenous delivery (Risner & Jones, 1980). It is as effective as cocaine in maintaining self-injection responding in squirrel monkeys, but is three to ten times less potent than cocaine (Spealman & Kelleher, 1981). Norcocaine is shorter acting than cocaine, which may account for the fact that it maintains high rates of responding across an entire session, even at the largest unit dose tested. The largest dose of cocaine, on the other hand, decreases response rates during the session (Spealman & Kelleher, 1981).

Because norcocaine probably does not reach effective levels in the body after the administration of cocaine, it is not likely that norcocaine is an essential product for any of the behavioral actions of administered cocaine. As noted by Spealman et al. (1979), biochemical studies have shown that norcocaine and cocaine are equipotent at inhibiting the reuptake of catecholamines in rat brain synaptosomes. If this should be true in other species as well, it would suggest that inhibition of catecholamine reuptake is not solely responsible for the behavioral effects of cocaine.

Endogenous Amines

Beta-phenylethylamine and phenylethanolamine, the noncatecholic analogs of dopamine and norepinephrine respectively, as well as other amines, are known to exist in trace amounts in the mammalian central nervous system. Some of these substances have been evaluated for their ability to initiate and maintain self-administration behavior in dogs under experimental conditions in which intravenous drug administration is contingent upon a single lever press. Both beta-phenylethylamine and phenylethanolamine are effective reinforcers in the dog; beta-phenylethylamine maintains a regularly spaced pattern of administration (Shannon & DeGregorio, 1982), similar to that reported for self-administration of cocaine.

Indirect evidence from drug discrimination experiments also suggests that endogenous amines may be important mediators of the discriminative stimulus effects of psychomotor stimulants. The ability of several MAO inhibitors to mimic the discriminative stimulus effects of cocaine in rats is highly correlated with their relative specificities for inhibiting type B MAO. Compounds that are relatively specific for type A MAO do not substitute for cocaine. One of the preferred endogenous substrates for type B MAO is phenethylamine, and phenethylamine substitutes for amphetamine as a discriminative stimulus under some experimental conditions (e.g., Huang & Ho, 1974c). Consequently, it has been argued (Colpaert et al., 1980) that endogenous substances other than dopamine, and perhaps phenethylamine, are most intimately involved in the discriminative stimulus effects of cocaine.

Dopamine Agonists

If the reinforcing effects of cocaine are mediated predominantly by dopamine receptor activation, other dopamine agonists should maintain self-administration behavior. Gill et al. (1978) demonstrated that apomorphine and piribedil maintain self-administration behavior in squirrel monkeys. Small doses of apomorphine appear to maintain behavior in some monkeys; larger doses produce erratic response rates and at some doses monkeys fail to respond. Woolverton et al. (1984) recently demonstrated that dopamine agonists (e.g., apomorphine, piribedil, propylbutyldopamine, bromocriptine) that act primarily on one type of dopamine receptor maintain self-administration in rhesus monkeys under fixed-ratio 10 schedules of reinforcement. Although all of the agonists of this type (DA2) tested do not maintain high rates of responding in all monkeys, each of them maintain high rates of responding in most of the monkeys. Cocaine, however, maintains high rates of responding in all monkeys. Each of these drugs has effects that are not related to dopamine, but the common effect of all these compounds is their dopamine agonist actions. A drug that acts primarily on DA1 receptors, SKF 38393, is not self-administered by monkeys. These investigators conclude that activation of DA2 receptors is most important for the reinforcing effects of these drugs. The drugs that are self-administered also produce increases in locomotor activity as do cocaine and d-amphetamine, and commonalities exist between patterns of cocaine and d-amphetamine self-administration and those of dopamine agonists.

DRUGS THAT MODIFY COCAINE-REINFORCED RESPONDING

As discussed earlier, the shape of the self-administration dose-rate curve is apparently determined by at least two effects of the drug: the reinforcing effect, reflected primarily in the increasing limb of the curve, and unconditioned effects of cocaine, reflected primarily in the decreasing limb of the curve. If a manipulation only decreases the reinforcing effect of cocaine, the ascending limb of the curve should be shifted to the right; the same manipulation should produce no change in the descending limb of the dose-effect curve. Procedures that decrease both reinforcing and unconditioned effects of cocaine would be expected to shift both limbs of the curve to the right. In the context of this simplified model of reinforcing and unconditioned effects of drugs that can act as positive reinforcers, it may be helpful to examine results from studies on possible modifications of the reinforcing effect of cocaine.

Studies of the effects of various drugs on the self-administration of cocaine are summarized in Table 2.4. Typically, only a single dose of cocaine was used in these studies, which means that effects on the complete cocaine-rate function, necessary to apply the analysis described above, cannot be determined. The most consistent finding of drug pretreatments on cocaine-maintained responding is that drugs such as chlorpromazine, haloperidol, and pimozide produce increases in the rate or amount of cocaine self-administration (Table

Table 2.4 Effects of Drug Pretreatment on Cocaine Self-Administration

Species	Pretreatment	Effect	Reference
Rat	Pimozide	INC	de Wit & Wise, 1977
	Phentolamine	DEC	de Wit & Wise, 1977
	Phenoxybenzamine	NE	de Wit & Wise, 1977
	Alpha-flupenthixol	INC	Ettenberg et al., 1982
	Naltrexone	NE	Ettenberg et al., 1982
	Sulpiride	INC	Roberts & Vickers, 1984
	Metoclopramide	INC	Roberts & Vickers, 1984
	Thioridazine	INC	Roberts & Vickers, 1984
	Chlorpromazine	INC	Roberts & Vickers, 1984
	Haloperidol	INC	Roberts & Vickers, 1984
	Flupenthixol	INC	Roberts & Vickers, 1984
	Clozapine	DEC	Roberts & Vickers, 1984
Rhesus monkey	Chlorpromazine	INC/DEC	Herling & Woods, 1980
	Haloperidol	INC	Woods et al., 1978
	Chlorpromazine	INC	Wilson & Schuster, 1972
	Atropine	INC	Wilson & Schuster, 1973b
	Methylatropine	NE	Wilson & Schuster, 1973b
	Physostigmine	DEC	Wilson & Schuster, 1973b
	AMPT	INC	Wilson & Schuster, 1974
	Pargyline	DEC	Wilson & Schuster, 1974
	Phentolamine	NE	Wilson & Schuster, 1974
	Phenoxybenzamine	NE	Wilson & Schuster, 1974
	Haloperidol	INC	de la Garza & Johanson, 1982
	Physostigmine	DEC	de la Garza & Johanson, 1982
	Perphenazine	INC	Johanson et al., 1976
	Pentobarbital	NE	Wilson & Schuster, 1973a
	Imipramine	NE	Wilson & Schuster, 1973a
	Morphine	NE	Wilson & Schuster, 1973a
	Propranolol	DEC	Golderg & Gonzalez, 1976
Squirrel monkey	Pimozide	INC	Gill et al., 1978
	Chlorpromazine	INC	Gill et al., 1978
	Chlordiazepoxide	NE	Gill et al., 1978
	Amitriptyline	NE	Gill et al., 1978
Dog	Phenoxybenzamine	NE	Risner & Jones, 1980
	Pimozide	INC	Risner & Jones, 1980
	Mecamylamine	NE	Risner & Goldberg, 1983

NE = no effect.
INC = increased response rate.
DEC = decreased response rate.

2.4). Although these drugs each have several pharmacological effects, they have in common the ability to antagonize dopamine receptor agonists. Other tested dopamine antagonists, including alpha-flupenthixol, sulpiride, metoclopramide, thioridazine, flupenthixol, and perphenazine also produce increases in cocaine self-administration; the only exception is clozapine, a dopamine receptor antagonist that produces only decreases in cocaine-maintained responding. Drugs that act as antagonists selectively at alpha adrenergic receptors do not alter cocaine self-administration. There are fewer studies of the effects of beta-adrenergic blockade on cocaine self-administration. Goldberg and Gonzalez (1976) find that propranolol, a beta-adrenergic antagonist, selectively decreases cocaine self-administration; doses of propanolol that decreased behavior maintained by cocaine do not alter similar rates of behavior maintained by food. Their data indicate that propranolol produces effects similar to those observed when the dose per injection of cocaine is increased.

The interaction between cholinergic antagonism and cocaine self-administration was evaluated by Wilson and Schuster (1973b). Atropine produces increases in cocaine self-administration, while methylatropine has no effect and physostimine produces decreases in cocaine self-administration.

These data indicate that antagonism of dopaminergic or cholinergic receptors produces increases in rates or amounts of self-administration of a single dose of cocaine, whereas antagonism of beta-adrenergic receptors or stimulation of cholinergic receptors produces decreases in cocaine-maintained behavior, and antagonism of alpha-adrenergic receptors has little effect. How have these various results been interpreted? Goldberg and Gonzalez attribute the propranolol-induced decrease in rates of cocaine self-administration to propranolol's effects on cardiac output. Decreases in cardiac output reduces blood flow to the liver which could result in decreased rates of cocaine metabolism and consequently increase the duration and effect of each dose of cocaine administered. The authors of the study investigating cholinergic influences on cocaine-maintained responding in monkeys suggest that atropine antagonizes the rate-decreasing effects of cocaine, but probably not the reinforcing effect of the drug.

Interestingly, very similar effects by dopamine antagonists on cocaine-maintained responding are typically interpreted as antagonism of cocaine's reinforcing effects. Many of the investigators who report that dopamine antagonists increase self-administration of cocaine, particularly those who study the effect in rats using FR 1 schedules of reinforcement, argue that these drugs antagonize specifically the reinforcing effects of cocaine. This argument is based on the observation that decreasing the unit dose of cocaine used to maintain behavior can lead to an increase in the number of cocaine injections the animals take. Thus, they suggest that administration of a dopamine antagonist effectively decreases the dose of cocaine, and a decrease in the effectiveness of a particular dose is tantamount to antagonizing the reinforcing effects of cocaine. There are two important flaws in this interpretation of the data. One is that cocaine dose-effect curves are rarely obtained prior to an evaluation of the effects of the pretreatment drugs, so it is not certain whether the dose of cocaine used to maintain the behavior is on the ascending or descending limb of the dose-effect curve. This is important because only if the cocaine dose is on the descending limb can one assume that an actual or effective decrease in the cocaine dose will lead to increases in cocaine intake. This point is critical, although the doses used in most studies were sufficiently large that they were almost certainly on the descending limb of the dose-effect curve. The second important point, rarely addressed or acknowledged by the investigators who interpret their results in terms of alterations of the reinforcing effect of cocaine, is that when doses on the descending limb of the cocaine unit dose-intake curve are evaluated, it is likely that the effect being measured involves more than the reinforcing effect of cocaine. The reinforcing effect at this point is accompanied by a strong rate-decreasing effect of cocaine. Therefore, when rates of cocaine self-administration are increased by presession administration of another drug, this might indicate only that the rate-decreasing effects of cocaine have been antagonized.

These criticisms of many studies on the effects of other drugs on cocaine self-administration are supported by data from a study by Herling and Woods (1980). In this experiment, behavior is maintained by one of several doses of cocaine under a second-order schedule of reinforcement. In a separate group of monkeys, responding is maintained under the same schedule of reinforcement by the delivery of food. When behavior is maintained by small doses of cocaine or by food, chlorpromazine produces only decreases in rates of responding. As shown in Figure 2.10, as the reinforcing dose of

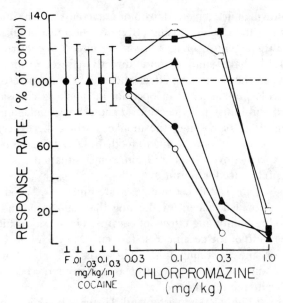

FIGURE 2.10. Antagonistic actions of chlorpromazine in rhesus monkeys trained to respond on a second-order fixed-interval 5-minute, fixed-ratio 10 [FI5 (FR10:S)] schedule of food or i.v. cocaine delivery. Abscissae: chlorpromazine dose in mg/kg. Ordinates: rate of responding expressed as a percentage of the response rate during saline pretreatment sessions. Solid circles represent food-reinforced responding. Cocaine-reinforced responding is represented by open circles (0.01 mg/kg/injection), triangles (0.03 mg/kg/injection), closed squares (0.1 mg/kg/injection), and open squares (0.3 mg/kg/injection). (From Herling & Woods, 1980)

cocaine is increased, chlorpromazine pretreatments result in increased rates of cocaine-maintained responding. Although chlorpromazine appears to decrease the effective dose of cocaine, the authors note that this very possibly had little to do with modification of the reinforcing effects of cocaine. It is more likely that chlorpromazine is antagonizing the behavioral effects of cocaine which alter rates and patterns of responding, and does not affect the reinforcing event. They noted that cocaine antagonizes the rate-decreasing effects of chlorpromazine and this reciprocal antagonism is also, in part, responsible for the increased rates of cocaine-reinforced responding.

This study indicates that increased rates of cocaine self-administration following injection of a dopamine antagonist may be due to an attenuation of the rate-decreasing effects of cocaine and not necessarily to an antagonism of its reinforcing effect. Woolverton and Balster (1981) have studied more directly effects of dopamine antagonists on the reinforcing effect of cocaine. These investigators evaluated chlorpromazine or haloperidol in monkeys choosing between food and infusions of cocaine. If these agents antagonize the reinforcing effect of cocaine, the monkeys would be expected to switch their choices from cocaine to food. In fact, animals continue to select cocaine over food and, in some situations, show an increased preference for cocaine.

By using an analysis of cocaine dose-rate functions, Woods et al. (1978) also provided evidence indicating that haloperidol does not antagonize the reinforcing effects of cocaine. Haloperidol shifts the descending limb of the cocaine dose-rate curve to the right, but has no effect on the ascending limb. These data clearly show that haloperidol antagonizes the rate-decreasing effects of cocaine, but fails to alter its reinforcing effect.

While the studies of Woolverton and Balster (1981) and Woods et al. (1978) suggest that dopamine antagonists do not influence the reinforcing effect of cocaine, other data indicate that these antagonists may alter the rate-increasing or reinforcing effects of cocaine. The interpretation of one such study is based on the premise that intermediate doses of dopamine antagonists should attenuate partially the reinforcing effects of cocaine and large doses of dopamine antagonists should antagonize completely the reinforcing effects of cocaine. Therefore, following administration of large doses of the antagonists, self-administration of cocaine should resemble the substitution of saline for cocaine. De Wit and Wise (1977) evaluated the effects of pimozide on cocaine self-administration in rats and find effects that may support this premise. As shown in Figure 2.11, intermediate doses of pimozide produce sustained increases in rate of cocaine-reinforced responding over time, presumably by antagonizing partially the effects of cocaine. Smaller doses of cocaine result in a similar increase in the rate of cocaine self-administration. More critical to their hypothesis are the data obtained with larger doses of pimozide, which produce a transient increase in cocaine-reinforced responding followed by a prolonged reduction in responding. The time course of this effect is similar to that observed when saline is substituted for cocaine. This

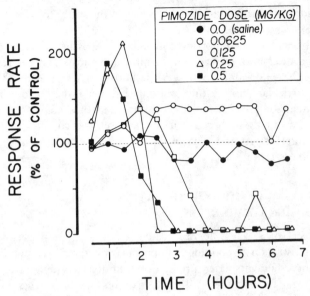

FIGURE 2.11. The effects of pimozide on behavior maintained by a fixed-ratio 1 schedule of intravenous cocaine (1.0 mg/kg/injection) self-administration in rats. Saline or pimozide (doses indicated by inset) was administered i.p. prior to test observations. Each point represents the median response rate for each dose group per half hour, expressed as a percentage of the control (i.e., no pretreatment) response rate. Abscissae: time in hours. (Modified from de Wit & Wise, 1977)

effect of pimozide is interpreted as a total antagonism of the reinforcing effect of cocaine. A similar effect would be expected, however, if pimozide were directly suppressing responding. In addition, a comparison of different schedules of reinforcement would be helpful if the schedules yield different time courses of rate decreases when saline is substituted. An evaluation of the effects of these doses of pimozide on behavior maintained by other reinforcers could also help clarify these data.

Herling (1980), using a dose-rate analysis of cocaine self-administration in the monkey, shows that chlorpromazine shifted the ascending limb of a cocaine dose-rate curve down and to the right while leaving the descending limb of this curve relatively unaffected. This result suggests a specific effect of chlorpromazine on the reinforcing effect of cocaine and is opposite to the effects shown with haloperidol on cocaine dose-rate functions in the study by Woods et al. (1978).

Clearly, with data supporting both sides of the issue regarding the presumed interaction between dopamine antagonists and the reinforcing effect of cocaine, there is no definitive answer at hand. The issue is particularly interesting, not only because it may help in the development of pharmacological treatment methodologies for cocaine abuse, but also because it underscores the complexities of experimental design and data interpretation that are necessary to resolve the question.

SCHEDULES OF COCAINE PRESENTATION AND COCAINE TERMINATION

The effects of a schedule of cocaine delivery upon patterns of self-administration responding may produce low rates of responding while only moments later produce extraordinarily high rates of responding. To encompass the description of the effects of a schedule of reinforcement requires a thorough knowledge of the immediate history and the exact nature of the schedule of cocaine delivery.

The complexity of schedule-controlled responding can be even greater. The same event—a schedule of cocaine delivery—can maintain a response that leads to its delivery while concurrently maintaining another response that leads to its termination. Spealman (1979) has carried out such an experiment with intravenous cocaine delivery in squirrel monkeys (Fig. 2.12). One response leads to the intermittent delivery of cocaine while a concurrently operating schedule leads to the termination of cocaine delivery for a short period. Figure 2.12 shows that over a range of doses, from the minimally effective dose to the optimal rate-maintaining dose, both types of schedules maintain behavior. If cocaine is eliminated, the responding controlled by both schedules is reduced. Further, if the schedules associated with the two responses are reversed, the patterns of responding reverse as well. Removing the termination contingency on the second lever results in a reduced rate of responding on this lever while responding on the first (i.e., cocaine-reinforced) lever is maintained. It thus seems clear that responding on the second lever is maintained by contingencies that eliminated the opportunity for cocaine self-administration. Spealman concludes

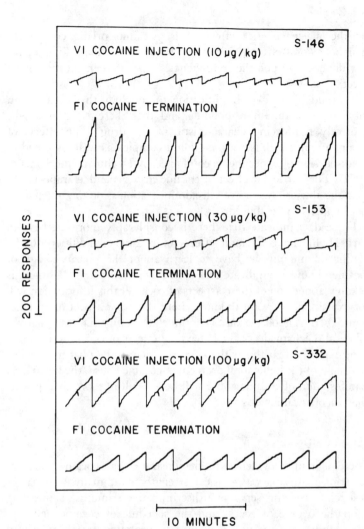

FIGURE 2.12. Characteristic response rates and temporal response patterns maintained simultaneously by cocaine injections and by terminating the schedule of cocaine injection. Responses on the right lever (upper record in each panel) produced intravenous injections of cocaine under a variable-interval (VI) schedule; responses on the left lever (lower record in each panel) terminated the schedule of cocaine injection for 1 minute under a fixed-interval (FI) schedule. Abscissae: time. Ordinates: cumulative number of lever presses. Diagonal marks in upper records indicate injections of cocaine. (From Spealman, 1979)

that the pharmacological effects of drugs cannot predict completely their behavioral effects, since these latter effects may differ markedly depending upon the contingencies of reinforcement that are in effect.

It would be an oversimplification to conclude that cocaine can only act to maintain responding and that there is an inherent, positively reinforcing characteristic of the drug. The effects of cocaine upon the abuser are no doubt complex as well, as noted in the discussion of experiments conducted by Fischman and Schuster (1982). The particular effect of cocaine may depend as importantly upon the abuser's history of self-administration as on the actual drug that happens to be abused.

These data indicate that there is considerably more we have to learn about the behavioral effects of cocaine in addition to the significant amount we have to learn about the pharmacology of cocaine. They also indicate that even if we should know all there is to know about one of these aspects of cocaine, this information will not explain all we want to know about the other aspect of cocaine. While there is good reason to continue an inquiry into the pharmacological mechanisms of the behavioral effects of cocaine, since it is to be expected that this is the best approach to the pharmacological treatment of the behavioral problem of cocaine abuse, the behavioral manifestation of cocaine abuse will be a result of more than just its pharmacological actions.

CONCLUSIONS

There is ample evidence to demonstrate that cocaine modifies behavior in striking ways—it can strengthen and maintain behavior as a reinforcer and serve as a discriminative stimulus. Depending upon the degree of access and the schedule of cocaine delivery, self-administered cocaine may lead to profound forms of central stimulation, including toxicity. When dose preferences are evaluated, there is a preference for larger doses of cocaine that appears limited only by toxicity. In some circumstances involving self-administration, drug discrimination, and the assessment of subjective effects, there are similarities between some of the local anesthetics and cocaine; thus, this action of cocaine may participate in some of its behavioral effects. Furthermore, cocaine shares some behavioral actions with dopamine releasers and dopamine receptor agonists. In addition, cocaine's behavioral actions are modified by dopamine receptor antagonists. These drugs antagonize many of the unconditioned actions of cocaine, but it is clear that at doses which reduce the discriminative stimulus and reinforcing effects of cocaine, the dopamine receptor antagonists that have been studied to date reduce many other behaviors as well. Certainly dopamine receptor antagonists are not likely to be effective in the treatment of cocaine abuse in the same way that narcotic antagonists are effective in the treatment of narcotic abuse, although they may have clinical usefulness in treating cocaine overdose. Perhaps because of the nature of the dopamine system and perhaps because we have not yet developed an ideal dopamine antagonist, these drugs have many unconditioned effects of their own that would preclude their chronic use as prophylactics.

REFERENCES

Aigner, T.G., Balster, R.L. (1978) Choice behavior in rhesus monkeys: cocaine versus food. *Science* 201:534–535.

Ando, K., Yanagita, T. (1978) The discriminative stimulus properties of intravenously administered cocaine in rhesus monkeys. In Colpaert, F.C., and Rosecrans, J.A. (eds.), *Stimulus Properties of Drugs: Ten Years of Progress.* Amsterdam: Elsevier/North-Holland Biomedical, pp. 125–136.

Balster, R.L., Schuster, C.R. (1973) Fixed-interval schedule of cocaine reinforcement: effect of dose and infusion duration. *J. Exp. Anal. Behav.* 20:119–129.

Bedford, J.A., Borne, R.F., Wilson, M.C. (1980) Comparative behavioral profile of cocaine and norcocaine in rats and monkeys. *Pharmacol. Biochem. Behav.* 13:69–75.

Bedford, J.A., Nail, G.L., Borne, R.F., Wilson, M.C. (1981) Discriminative stimulus properties of cocaine, norcocaine, and n-allylnor-cocaine. *Pharmacol. Biochem. Behav.* 14:81–83.

Colpaert, F.C., Janssen, P.A.J. (1982) Factors regulating drug cue sensitivity: Limits of discriminability and the role of a progressively decreasing training dose in cocaine-saline discrimination. *Neuropharmacol.* 21:1187–1194.

Colpaert, F.C., Niemegeers, C.J.E., Janssen, P.A.J. (1980) Evidence that a preferred substrate for type B monoamine oxidase mediates stimulus properties of MAO inhibitors: a possible role for beta-phenyl-ethylamine in the cocaine cue. *Pharmacol. Biochem. Behav.* 13:513–517.

Colpaert, F.C., Niemegeers, C.J.E., Janssen, P.A.J. (1979) Discriminative stimulus properties of cocaine: neuropharmacological characteristics as derived from stimulus generalization experiments. *Pharmacol. Biochem. Behav.* 10:535–546.

Colpaert, F.C., Niemegeers, C.J.E., Janssen, P.A.J. (1978) Discriminative stimulus properties of cocaine and d-amphetamine, and antagonism by haloperidol: A comparative study. *Neuropharmacol.* 17:937–942.

Colpaert, F.C., Niemegeers, C.J.E., Janssen, P.A.J. (1976) Cocaine cue in rats as it relates to subjective drug effects: a preliminary report. *Eur. J. Pharmacol.* 40:195–199.

Cunningham, K.A., Appel, J.B. (1982) Discriminative stimulus properties of cocaine and phencyclidine: similarities in the mechanism of action. In Colpaert, F.C. and Slangen, J.L. (eds.), *Drug Discrimination: Applications in CNS Pharmacology.* Amsterdam: Elsevier Biomedical Press, pp. 181–192.

Deneau, G., Yanagita, T., Seevers, M.H. (1969) Self-administration of psychoactive substances by the monkey: a measure of psychological dependence. *Psychopharmacol.* 16:30–48.

Downs, D.A., Woods, J.H. (1974) Codeine- and cocaine-reinforced responding in rhesus monkeys: effects of dose on response rates under a fixed-ratio schedule. *J. Pharmacol. Exp. Ther.* 191:179–188.

D'Mello, G.D., Stolerman, I.P. (1977) Comparison of the discriminative stimulus properties of cocaine and amphetamine in rats. *Br. J. Pharmacol.* 61:415–422.

de la Garza, R., Johanson, C.E. (1985) Discriminative stimulus properties of cocaine in pigeons. *Psychopharmacol.* 85:23–30.

de la Garza, R., Johanson, C.E. (1983) The discriminative stimulus properties of cocaine in the rhesus monkey. *Pharmacol. Biochem. Behav.* 19:145–148.

de la Garza, R., Johanson, C.E. (1982) Effects of haloperidol and physostigmine on self-administration of local anesthetics. *Pharmacol. Biochem. Behav.* 17:1295–1299.

De Wit, H., Wise, R.A. (1977) Blockade of cocaine reinforcement in rats with the dopamine receptor blocker pimozide, but not with the noradrenergic blockers phentolamine or phenoxybenzamine. *Canad. J. Psychol.* 31:195–203.

Ettenberg, A., Pettit, H.O., Bloom, F.E., Koob, G.F. (1982) Heroin and cocaine intravenous self-administration in rats: mediation by separate neural systems. *Psychopharmacol.* 78:204–209.

Fischman, M.W., Schuster, C.R. (1982) Cocaine self-administration in humans. *Fed. Proc.* 41:241–246.

Fischman, M.W., Schuster, C.R. (1983a) A comparison of the subjective and cardiovascular effects of cocaine and lidocaine in humans. *Pharmacol. Biochem. Behav.* 18:123–127.

Fischman, M.W., Schuster, C.R., Rajfer, S. (1983b) A comparison of the subjective and cardiovascular effects of cocaine and procaine in humans. *Pharmacol. Biochem. Behav.* 18:711–716.

Fischman, M.W., Schuster, C.R., Resnekov, L., Shick, J.F.E., Krasnegor, N.A., Fennell, W., Freedman, D.X. (1976) Cardiovascular and subjective effects of intravenous cocaine administration in humans. *Arch. Gen. Psychiat.* 33:983–989.

Ford, R.D., Balster, R.L. (1977) Reinforcing properties of intravenous procaine in rhesus monkeys. *Pharmacol. Biochem. Behav.* 6:289–295.

Gill, C.A., Holz, W.C., Zirkle, C.L., Hill, H. (1978) Pharmacological modification of cocaine and apomorphine self-administration in the squirrel monkey. *Proceedings of the 10th Congress of the Collegium Internationale Neuro-Psychopharmacologicum.* 2:1477–1484.

Goldberg, S.R., Gonzalez, F.A. (1976) Effects of propranolol on behavior maintained under fixed-ratio schedules of cocaine injection or food presentation in squirrel monkeys. *J. Pharmacol. Exp. Ther.* 198: 626–634.

Griffith, J.D. (1977) Amphetamine dependence; clinical factors. In Martin, W.R. (ed.), *Drug Addiction II: Amphetamine, Psychotogen, and Marihuana Dependence, Handbuch der Experimentellen Pharmakologie,* Vol. 45, No. 2. Berlin: Springer-Verlag, pp. 277–303.

Griffith, J.D., Cavanaugh, J., Held, J., Oates, J.A. (1972) Dextroamphetamine: evaluation of psychomimetic properties in men. *Arch. Gen. Psychiat.* 26:97–100.

Griffiths, R.R., Bradford, L.D., Brady, J.V. (1979) Progressive-ratio and fixed-ratio schedules of cocaine-maintained responding in baboons. *Psychopharmacol.* 65:125–136.

Griffiths, R.R., Brady, J.V., Snell, J.D. (1978) Progressive-ratio performance maintained by drug infusions: comparison of cocaine, diethylpropion, chlorphentermine, and fenfluramine. *Psychopharmacol.* 56:5–13.

Hammberbeck, D.M., Mitchell, C.L. (1978) The reinforcing properties of procaine and d-amphetamine compared in rhesus monkeys. *J. Pharmacol. Exp. Ther.* 204:558–569.

Herling, S. (1980) An analysis of specificity of drug-induced changes in drug-reinforced responding. Ph.D. dissertation, University of Michigan Medical School.

Herling, S., Woods, J.H. (1980) Chlorpromazine effects on cocaine-reinforced responding in rhesus monkeys: reciprocal modification of rate-altering effects of the drugs. *J. Pharmacol. Exp. Ther.* 214:354–361.

Herling, S., Downs, D.A., Woods, J.H. (1979) Cocaine, d-amphetamine, and pentobarbital effects on responding maintained by food or cocaine in rhesus monkeys. *Psychopharmacol.* 64:261–269.

Ho, B.T., Huang, J.-T. (1975) Role of dopamine in d-amphetamine-induced discriminative responding. *Pharmacol. Biochem. Behav.* 3:1085–1092.

Ho, B.T., McKenna, M. (1978) Discriminative stimulus properties of central stimulants. In Ho, B.T., Richards, D.W., III and Chute, D.L. (eds.), *Drug Discrimination and State Dependent Learning.* New York: Academic Press, pp. 67–77.

Huang, J.-T., Ho, B.T. (1974a) Discriminative stimulus properties of d-amphetamine and related compounds in rats. *Pharmacol. Biochem. Behav.* 2:669–673.

Huang, J.-T., Ho, B.T. (1974b) Effects of nikethamide, picrotoxin and strychnine on "amphetamine state." *Eur. J. Pharmacol.* 29:175–178.

Huang, J.-T., Ho, B.T. (1974c) The effect of pretreatment with iproniazid on the behavioral activities of beta-phenylethylamine in rats. *Psychopharmacol.* 35:77–81.

Iglauer, C., Woods, J.H. (1974) Concurrent performances: reinforcement by different doses of intravenous cocaine in rhesus monkeys. *J. Exp. Anal. Behav.* 22:179–196.

Jarbe, T.U.C. (1981) Cocaine cue in pigeons: Time course studies and generalization to structurally related compounds (norcocaine, WIN 35,428 and 35,065–2) and (+)-amphetamine. *Br. J. Pharmacol.* 73:843–852.

Jarbe, T.U.C. (1978) Cocaine as a discriminative cue in rats: interactions with neuroleptics and other drugs. *Psychopharmacol.* 59:183–187.

Jasinski, D.E., Nutt, J.G., Griffith, J.D. (1974) Effects of diethylproprion and d-amphetamine after subcutaneous and oral administration. *Clin. Pharmacol. Therap.* 16:645–652.

Johanson, C. (1980) The reinforcing properties of procaine, chloroprocaine and proparacaine in rhesus monkeys. *Psychopharmacol.* 67:189–194.

Johanson, C.E., Aigner, T. (1981) Comparison of the reinforcing properties of cocaine and procaine in rhesus monkeys. *Pharmacol. Biochem. Behav.* 15:49–53.

Johanson, C.E., Schuster, C.R. (1975) A choice procedure for drug reinforcers: cocaine and methylphenidate in the rhesus monkey. *J. Pharmacol. Exp. Ther.* 193:676–688.

Johanson, C.E., Kandel, D.A., Bonese, K. (1976) The effects of perphenazine on self-administration behavior. *Pharmacol. Biochem. Behav.* 4:427–433.

Martin, W.R., Sloan, J.W., Sapira, J.D., Jasinski, D.R. (1971) Physiologic, subjective, and behavioral effects of amphetamine, methamphetamine, ephedrine, phenmetrazine, and methylphenidate in man. *Clin. Pharmacol. Ther.* 12:245–258.

McKenna, M.L., Ho, B.T. (1980) The role of dopamine in the discriminative stimulus properties of cocaine. *Neuropharmacol.* 19:297–303.

McKenna, M.L., Ho, B.T., Englert, L.F. (1979) Generalization of norcocaine to the discriminative stimulus properties of cocaine. *Pharmacol. Biochem. Behav.* 10:273–276.

Pickens, R., Thompson, T. (1968) Cocaine-reinforced behavior in rats: effects of reinforcement magnitude and fixed-ratio size. *J. Pharmacol. Exp. Ther.* 161:122–129.

Richards, D.W., III, Harris, R.T., Ho, B.T. (1973) Central control of d-amphetamine-induced discriminative stimuli. Abstract, 3rd Annual Meeting, Society for Neuroscience, San Diego.

Risner, M.E., Goldberg, S.R. (1983) A comparison of nicotine and cocaine self-administration in the dog: fixed-ratio and progressive-ratio schedules of intravenous drug infusion. *J. Pharmacol. Exp. Ther.* 224:319–326.

Risner, M.E., Jones, B.E. (1980) Intravenous self-administration of cocaine and norcocaine by dogs. *Psychopharmacol.* 71:83–89.

Roberts, D.C.S., Vickers, G. (1984) Atypical neuroleptics increase self-administration of cocaine: an evaluation of a behavioural screen for antipsychotic activity. *Psychopharmacol.* 82:135–139.

Schechter, M.D., Cook, P.G. (1975) Dopaminergic mediation of the interoceptive cue produced by d-amphetamine in rats. *Psychopharmacol.* 42:185–193.

Schechter, M.D., Rosecrans, J.A. (1972) d-amphetamine as a discriminative cue: drugs with similar stimulus properties. *Psychopharmacol.* 21:212–216.

Shannon, H.E., DeGregorio, C.M. (1982) Self-administration of the endogenous trace amines beta-phenylethylamine, n-methyl phenylethylamine and phenylethanolamine in dogs. *J. Pharmacol. Exp. Ther.* 222:52–60.

Silverman, P.B., Ho, B.T. (1977) Characterization of discriminative response control by psychomotor stimulants. In Lal, H. (ed.), *Advances in Behavioral Biology*, Vol. 22, *Discriminative Stimulus Properties of Drugs*. New York: Plenum Press, pp. 107–119.

Spealman, R.D. (1979) Behavior maintained by termination of a schedule of self-administered cocaine. *Science* 204:1231–1232.

Spealman, R.D., Kelleher, R.T. (1981) Self-administration of cocaine derivatives by squirrel monkeys. *J. Pharmacol. Exp. Ther.* 216:532–536.

Spealman, R.D., Kelleher, R.T. (1979) Behavioral effects of self-

administered cocaine: responding maintained alternately by cocaine
and electric shock in squirrel monkeys. *J. Pharmacol. Exp. Ther.*
210:206–214.

Spealman, R.D., Goldberg, S.R., Kelleher, R.T., Morse W.H., Goldberg,
D.M., Hakansson, C.G., Nieforth, K.A., Lazer, E.S. (1979) Effects
of norcocaine and some norcocaine derivatives on schedule-
controlled behavior of pigeons and squirrel monkeys. *J. Pharmacol.
Exp. Ther.* 210:196–705.

Spealman, R.D., Kelleher, R.T., Goldberg, R. (1983) Stereoselective
behavioral effects of cocaine and a phenyltropane analog. *J.
Pharmacol. Exp. Ther.* 225:509–514.

Van Dyke, C., Jatlow, P., Ungerer, J., Barash, P., Byck, R. (1978)
Comparative psychological effects after intranasal application of local
anesthetics: lidocaine and cocaine. In *Problems of Drug Dependence
1978. Proceedings of the 40th Annual Scientific Meeting.* Committee on
Problems of Drug Dependence, pp. 322–332.

Wallach, M.B., Gershon, S. (1972) The induction and antagonism of
central nervous system stimulant-induced stereotyped behavior in
the cat. *Eur. J. Pharmacol.* 18:22–26.

Wilson, M.C., Schuster, C.R. (1974) Aminergic influences on intravenous
cocaine self-administration by rhesus monkeys. *Pharmacol. Biochem.
Behav.* 2:563–571.

Wilson, M.C., Schuster, C.R. (1973a) The effects of stimulants and
depressants on cocaine self-administration in the rhesus monkey.
Psychopharmacol. 31:291–304.

Wilson, M.C., Schuster, C.R. (1973b) Cholinergic influence on intravenous
cocaine self-administration by rhesus monkeys. *Pharm. Biochem.
Behav.* 1:643–649.

Wilson, M.C., Schuster, C.R. (1972) The effects of chlorpromazine on
psychomotor stimulant self-administration in the rhesus monkey.
Psychopharmacol. 26:115–126.

Wilson, M.C., Hitomi, M., Schuster, C.R. (1971) Psychomotor-stimulant
self-administration as a function of dosage per injection in the rhesus
monkey. *Psychopharmacol.* 22:271–281.

Winger, G.D., Woods, J.H. (1985) Comparison of fixed-ratio and
progressive-ratio schedules of maintenance of stimulant drug-
reinforced responding. *Drug Alc. Depend.* 15:123–130.

Woods, J.H., Herling, S., Winger, G. (1978) Chlorpromazine- and
haloperidol-induced changes in some behavioral effects of cocaine
and amphetamine. *Proceedings of the 10th Congress,* Collegium
Internationale Neuro-psychopharmacologicum, 2:1485–1502.

Woolverton, W.L., Balster, R.L. (1983) Effects of local anesthetics on fixed-interval responding in rhesus monkeys. *Pharmacol. Biochem. Behav.* 18:383–387.

Woolverton, W.L., Balster, R.L. (1981) Effects of antipsychotic compounds in rhesus monkeys given a choice between cocaine and food. *Drug Alc. Depend.* 8:69–78.

Woolverton, W.L., Balster, R.L. (1979) Reinforcing properties of some local anesthetics in rhesus monkeys. *Pharmacol. Biochem. Behav.* 11:669–672.

Woolverton, W.L., Goldberg, L.I., Ginos, J.Z. (1984) Intravenous self-administration of dopamine receptor agonists by rhesus monkeys. *J. Pharmacol. Exp. Ther.* 230:678–683.

3 | Neuronal Bases for Hedonic Effects of Cocaine and Opiates

CONAN KORNETSKY and GEORGE BAIN

THE THESIS that we will present in this chapter is that opioids and central nervous system stimulants share a common central mechanism that subserves the hedonic effect of these drugs. Further, this hedonic effect is the primary determinant of their abuse. Most theories concerned with why people abuse drugs are based on the hypothesis that the individual is psychologically or biologically deviant. An example is the writings of Khantzian (1980), who argued that "opiates counteracted regressed, disorganized, and dysphoric ego states associated with overwhelming feelings of rage, anger and related depression." Dole and Nyswander (1967), in introducing the use of methadone to treat heroin addiction, argued that there is a metabolic disturbance in the narcotic addict and that drug use is restorative.

The replacement or return-to-normality hypotheses are persuasive. Certainly a depressed person might find cocaine or heroin helpful in relieving depression. However, there would be little abuse if these substances did not cause some feeling of well-being or euphoria beyond simple restoration of a normal state—otherwise we would have abuse problems with almost every therapeutic drug, and we do not. Although abuse of drugs cannot be explained by a single causative factor, we would argue that for many drugs a necessary ingredient of their nonmedical use is that they will cause a feeling of euphoria and well-being, and this may be sufficient reinforcement so that drug-seeking behavior is engendered. The question we will address in this chapter is whether the euphoria caused by CNS stimulants (i.e., cocaine and d-amphetamine) and the opioids have some common central neuronal mediation. Experiments from our laboratory (Esposito et al., 1978; Kornetsky et al., 1979) suggest that this common action of these abuse substances is, at the level of the CNS, manifested as an activation of those areas of the brain for which electrical stimulation is rewarding. For the user, the activation of these reward areas of the brain is translated into some pleasurable feelings that are often described as the "high." In an animal the effect is sufficiently reinforcing that the animal will press levers in order to receive the drug or the drug will make the animal more sensitive to rewarding brain stimulation.

The suggestion that abuse substances achieve their reinforcing properties by activation of a reward system in the brain was suggested not too many years after the seminal discovery by Olds and Milner (1954) that rats will work in order to receive electrical stimulation to certain brain sites. This phenomenon has been called intracranial self-stimulation (ICSS) and more recently the term brain-stimulation reward has been added. For the most part, the former term has been employed when the animals are in an operant paradigm in which the dependent variable is rate of response (usually lever pressing).

In 1956 Olds et al. reported on the effects of chlorpromazine and reserpine on ICSS and in 1957 Killam and colleagues presented a paper at a meeting of the American Society for Pharmacology and Experimental Therapeutics reporting that 10 mg/kg of pentobarbital caused a slight increase in rate of response in rats with stimulating electrodes in some, but not all, areas of the hypothalamus. They also reported that amphetamine increased rate of response and probably lowered the stimulation threshold for rewarding brain stimulation.

Despite these interesting early studies, there was not a great deal of interest in the use of rewarding brain stimulation as a method for the study of the rewarding effects of opioids or the CNS stimulants. In 1960 Olds and Travis reported on the effects of morphine on ICSS. After this 1960 paper we could find no published reports on the effects of opiates on ICSS until a report by Adams et al. in 1972. During this period there was little interest in the effects of amphetamine (Stark et al., 1969; Stein & Ray, 1960; Stein, 1962, 1964) or cocaine (Stein, 1962; Benesova, 1969; Crow, 1970), although most of these investigators found that these two drugs facilitate self-stimulation. The failure to evaluate the action of abuse substances on ICSS, with the exceptions noted above, was probably not surprising, considering the early equivocal results obtained with morphine

(Olds & Travis, 1960). Also, in 1962 Weeks described an experiment in which he was able to train rats to lever press for morphine delivered by means of an indwelling venous catheter. The obvious homologous nature of this model resulted in a flurry of research activity that eclipsed other models of drug abuse. Further, the 1960s saw the emergence of the use of drugs as discriminative stimuli (Overton, 1964), which took precedence over the less understandable ICSS procedure.

The drug self-administration procedure clearly had face validity for the study of abuse substances, and the drugs as discriminative stimuli method is, in many ways, an animal analogue of the NIDA Addiction Research Center's method of determining the abuse potential of new compounds in humans. Although both of these methods are useful, as originally employed they do not tell us anything about the neuronal basis for the reinforcing effect of a drug—only whether or not it is reinforcing or whether or not a drug has effects similar to known abuse substances. It should be pointed out, however, that recently there have been systematic studies in which the neuronal systems were manipulated in order to determine the role of specific brain sites or systems in drug self-administration (Ettenberg et al., 1982; Pettit et al., 1984).

We first looked at the effects of opiates on rewarding brain stimulation in the early 1970s (Marcus & Kornetsky, 1974). Since we believed that the important question was whether morphine changed the threshold for rewarding brain stimulation and not whether rate of response for rewarding brain stimulation was altered, we directly measured the absolute threshold. This experiment was the first classical psychophysical study of ICSS that measured the threshold in a rate (of response) free paradigm. Absolute threshold was defined as the intensity of stimulation at which half the time the animal found it reinforcing and half the time nonreinforcing. As expected, we found a clear lowering of the reward threshold after morphine. This increase in sensitivity to the rewarding stimulation was not seen at higher doses (10 mg/kg) so that the dose-effect curve was U shaped. Subsequently, we have found that every drug that lowers the reward threshold has a U-shaped dose-response curve if sufficient doses are tested.

Since the Marcus and Kornetsky (1974) experiment we have studied a number of abuse substances and have found no false positives. That is, every substance that lowers the threshold for rewarding brain stimulation is abused by humans or has the potential for abuse as determined by independent assays. For example, we found that tripelennamine, an antihistamine, will slightly but significantly lower the threshold (Unterwald et al., 1984a) for rewarding brain stimulation, and Jasinski et al. (1983) found that human subjects report an euphoria after intramuscular administration. Although we have thus far found no false positives, there are abused substances that only raise the threshold. These seem to be the sedative hypnotics (e.g., alcohol) (Unterwald et al., 1984b) and pentobarbital (unpublished data).

Our findings that cocaine (Esposito et al., 1978) and amphetamine (Esposito et al., 1980) will lower the threshold in a manner similar to that of the opiates, including heroin (Hubner & Kornetsky, 1984), led us to postulate that euphoria caused by these drugs may be mediated by a common neuronal mechanism. This is not to say that the euphoria produced by cocaine is the same as that of heroin. Certainly the human drug user can tell the difference between heroin and cocaine and so can animals in drug discrimination experiments. However, the underlying mechanisms involved may be similar but the manner in which these neuronal changes express themselves at the conscious level may differ. Each drug has other actions that also shape the final effect experienced by the subject.

Although cocaine and heroin may cause similar effects on some measure, this does not prove that there is a common mechanism of action. We can reduce the ability of an animal to make a simple visual discrimination by administering a high dose of a drug as well as by destroying the optic nerve, but despite a similarity in the effects of these two maneuvers, we have not found a common mechanism. A more specific test would be whether or not a specific competitive antagonist that has no effect of its own would block the threshold-lowering effect of both morphine and cocaine.

If there is a common neuronal substrate for the effects of those drugs that increase the sensitivity of the animal to rewarding brain stimulation, then the obvious system is that which subserves ICSS behavior. Most investigators have argued that the underlying neurochemical substrate for rewarding brain stimulation is catecholaminergic with emphasis on the dopamine system (e.g., Fibiger, 1978; Wise & Bozarth, 1982; Gallistel et al., 1981; Olds & Forbes, 1981). More recently, however, Prado-Alcala and Wise (1984) and Prado-Alcala et al. (1984) found that there is not a close correspondence between the boundaries of the brain-reward system and those of the dopamine terminal fields. These findings suggest that a direct activation of a dopaminergic system does not account for the rewarding effects of stimulation to a variety of brain sites.

A suggestion that histamine may play a role is the finding by Unterwald et al. (1984a) that the antihistamine tripelennamine will lower the threshold for rewarding brain stimulation and potentiate the threshold-lowering effect of pentazocine (Unterwald & Kornetsky, 1984), a mixed opiate agonist-antagonist. Although antihistamine drugs have other actions besides blocking the release of histamine, (e.g., anticholinergic, local anesthetic), we have found that the anticholinergics scopolamine, atropine, and trihexphenidyl as well as the local anesthetic procaine do not lower the reward threshold (unpublished data). Thus, it is unlikely that the tripelennamine effect on rewarding brain stimulation is a result of these nonantihistaminic actions of this drug. However, we did find that scopolamine or atropine, at relatively high doses, will decrease the sensitivity of the animal to rewarding brain stimulation. This is in agreement with a postulated cholinergic modulation of brain-stimulation rewards (Olds & Domino, 1969a, 1969b; Gratton & Wise, 1985).

Other investigators have postulated a role for an endorphin system in brain-stimulation reward. This hypothesis was first suggested by Belluzzi and Stein (1977). The involvement of an endogenous opiate system in brain-stimulation reward is based on their findings that naloxone will attenuate ICSS. Although other investigators also have found that naloxone will attenuate ICSS behavior (Stapleton et al., 1979; Schaefer & Michael, 1981), some investigators using similar procedures with electrodes in some of the same brain areas have failed to find that naloxone will alter ICSS (Wauquier et al., 1974; Holzman, 1976; van der Kooy et al., 1977; Lorens & Sainati, 1978). Stapleton et al. in their 1979 paper concluded that it took relatively large doses of naloxone to alter ICSS (10 mg/kg) but it did not abolish the behavior and only caused modest reduction in response rate. They concluded that although endorphinergic processes may modify reward, they do not seem critical for reward. We also have found that naloxone has no effect on the threshold for rewarding brain stimulation after both single doses (Esposito et al., 1980) and after daily administration (Perry et al., 1981).

Even if an endogenous opiate system is not critical for reward, it is still possible that the ability of cocaine, amphetamine, and the opiates to increase the sensitivity of an animal to rewarding brain stimulation may be a function of similar neuronal mechanisms. Although naloxone does not alter the sensitivity of an animal to rewarding brain stimulation, it will antagonize the threshold-lowering effect of morphine (Kornetsky & Wheeling, 1982). For example, we have found that the threshold-lowering effect of 2 mg/kg of morphine can be completely blocked by doses of naloxone as low as 0.05 mg/kg and partially blocked by 0.025 mg/kg. If naloxone could also alter the threshold-lowering effect of CNS stimulants, it would suggest a possible common mechanism for this aspect of the effects of opiates and cocaine or d-amphetamine.

This hypothesis was tested in two experiments. In the first, various doses of naloxone were combined with 0.5 or 1.0 mg/kg of d-amphetamine (Esposito et al., 1980). Both of these doses significantly lowered the threshold for rewarding brain stimulation. Although naloxone had no effect by itself except to increase intrasubject variability, a dose of 2.0 mg/kg or above blocked the threshold-lowering effect of d-amphetamine in each of four animals tested. An interesting phenomenon was observed in that at the highest dose of naloxone tested (16 mg/kg), two of the four animals showed a marked decrease in the ability of naloxone to block the d-amphetamine effect.

In the second study (Kornetsky & Bain, 1983) we compared the effects of cocaine in combination with naloxone. As in the previous study naloxone alone had no significant effects on the sensitivity of the animal. However, at doses of approximately 4 mg/kg naloxone blocked or attenuated the effect of cocaine. Figure 3.1 shows the effect of this combination in one of the six animals in this study. This was the typical pattern seen. As shown, 15 mg/kg of cocaine by itself lowers the threshold for rewarding brain stimulation. However, 4 mg/kg of naloxone significantly attentuated this effect. It is interesting to note that higher doses of naloxone were less effective in blocking the effects of cocaine. This suggests a possible narrow window of doses of naloxone that will attenuate the effects of the CNS stimulants.

Although naloxone attenuated the threshold-lowering effect of cocaine or d-amphetamine, it did this somewhat differently than when blocking the effect of morphine. The dose of naloxone needed

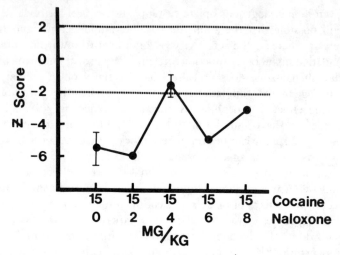

FIGURE 3.1. An example is shown of the effects in one subject of 15 mg/kg of cocaine alone and in combination with various doses of naloxone on the threshold for rewarding brain stimulation. Data are expressed as Z scores based on the mean and standard deviation of 16 saline test days. Negative scores indicate a lowering of the threshold-increased sensitivity. The dotted lines define the 95% confidence limits. Thus, points within these lines indicate effects not different from saline. Since doses of 15 mg/kg of cocaine alone and 15 mg/kg of cocaine plus 4 mg/kg of naloxone were repeated several times, the standard error of the mean Z score is indicated by the vertical lines.

to block a threshold-lowering dose of morphine is significantly lower than the doses necessary to block the effects of cocaine or d-amphetamine. Also, another difference was observed. When naloxone blocked the effects of morphine, it not only blocked the threshold-lowering effects but it blocked all the actions of this opiate. When naloxone blocked the effects of cocaine or d-amphetamine it blocked only the threshold-lowering effects of these drugs. Other CNS effects that we could observe appeared unaltered. The animals showed the same amount of psychomotor excitement as they did when receiving these CNS stimulant drugs alone. This is illustrated in Figure 3.2. Here a Venn diagram represents the effects of morphine and cocaine, with euphoria the only effect they have in common, and it is the effect blocked by naloxone.

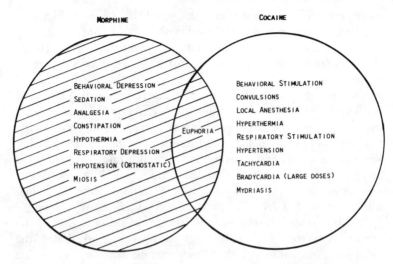

FIGURE 3.2. The effects of morphine are shown in the circle at the left and the effects of cocaine in the circle at the right. The area of overlap represents the common effect, euphoria, produced by both agents. The crosshatching indicates those effects of both agents that are reversed by naloxone.

Further evidence of the relationship between dopamine agonists and opiate drugs is the potentiation of the euphoric effect reported when cocaine and heroin, or d-amphetamine and heroin are concomitantly administered in humans. For example, Jasinski and Nutt (1972) gave various combinations of morphine and d-amphetamine to human subjects and found that the reported degree of euphoria was greater than that obtained with either drug alone. Hubner et al. (1983) demonstrated that the combination of these two drugs produced a lowering of the threshold for rewarding brain stimulation in the rat that also was greater than with either drug alone.

The interrelation between a catecholaminergic and an endorphinergic system is demonstrated in the finding that opiate receptors have been discovered on dopaminergic presynaptic neurons in both the mesolimbic system as well as the striatum (Pollard et al., 1977a, 1977b). It is believed that these opiate receptors serve to modulate dopamine synthesis and release.

Although earlier investigators have suggested that the role of the opiate receptor in modulating the release and turnover of dopamine is inhibitory (Pollard et al., 1977a, 1977b; Schwartz et al., 1978), more recently investigators have suggested the opposite (Biggio et al., 1978; Smith et al., 1980; Wood et al., 1980). Thus, combining opiate and dopamine agonists results in potentiation of the effect, while an opiate antagonist will attenuate the action of a dopamine agonist.

The finding that naloxone will attenuate the rewarding effects of cocaine or d-amphetamine without much effect on the psychomotor excitation effect suggests that there is a dissociation between the euphoria and psychomotor stimulant effects of these drugs. Further support for a common substrate for the rewarding effects of these compounds is the report that haloperidol will block morphine self-administration (Glick & Cox, 1975; Hanson & Cimini-Venema, 1972; Pozuelo & Kerr, 1972).

Despite the above findings, some contrary evidence is given in the report by Pettit et al. (1984) (see also Chapter 4). Using the self-administration model, they found that destruction of dopamine terminals in the nucleus accumbens of the rat by the direct application of 6-hydroxy-dopamine would selectively attenuate cocaine but not heroin self-administration. Although this finding would suggest that separate systems may subserve the rewarding effects of these drugs, it could also mean that there is not a one-to-one confirmation in the brain of the action of the opiates and the CNS stimulants on the reinforcing effects of these drugs. Also, there is the possibility that heroin self-administration is not only a result of the rewarding effects of the drug but other contingencies may drive the self-administration of heroin behavior. The most likely candidate is physical dependence.

Further evidence for the role of the reward system in mediating the action of drugs is the report by Seeger et al. (1984). This group used the quantitative 2-deoxyglucose method of Sokoloff (1982) to study the effects of amphetamine on rewarding brain stimulation. It is likely that the effects they observed with d-amphetamine would hold for cocaine. Animals were prepared with electrodes implanted in the ventral tegmental area (VTA). They compared four groups of animals: high current, low current plus 0.5 mg/kg of d-amphetamine, 0.5 mg/kg d-amphetamine but not allowed to self-stimulate, and a no treatment group. In the high current and low current plus amphetamine groups, response rates for rewarding stimulation were approximately the same. Rates of local cerebral glucose utilization (LCGU) was lower at the stimulation site and pathway in the low current plus *d*-amphetamine group than the high current group. However, in a number of the projection areas of the VTA, LCGU's were equivalent (i.e., the nucleus accumbens, the medial frontal cortex, the basolateral amygdala and the locus coeruleus). In the olfactory tubercle and the sulcal cortex, LCGU was greater in the low stimulation plus *d*-amphetamine group than in the high stimulation group.

Although these are some of the first drug-brain stimulation studies done by this group of investigators, the findings support the contention that abuse substances activate functional reward systems, and a reasonable assumption is that this may be the basis for the euphoric properties of both the opiates as well as the CNS stimulants.

Further, there is no need to postulate that drug abusers are necessarily psychologically or biologically deviant. Simple euphoria is probably sufficiently reinforcing to maintain the drug-seeking behavior. This is not to say that there are no deviant drug users, but it does suggest that treatment programs that assume the user is psychologically sick are not likely to affect a change in the drug-seeking behavior. Jaffe (1984) stated in a paper on the evaluation of drug abuse treatment that those subjects with the greatest amount of psychopathology were those least amenable to a treatment program aimed at obtaining drug-free clients. However, it does not follow from this that the psychopathology caused the drug abuse. Often ignored is the hedonic nature of humans and, whether or not psychopathology exists, hedonic pleasure will be pursued.

REFERENCES

Adams, W.J., Lorens, S.A., Mitchell, C.L. (1972) Morphine enhances lateral hypothalamic self-stimulation in the rat. *Proc. Soc. Exp. Biol.* 140:770–771.

Belluzzi, J.D., Stein, L. (1977) Enkephalin- and morphine-induced facilitation of long term memory. *Soc. Neurosci. Abst.* III:230.

Benesova, O. (1969) The action of cocaine, atropine, and tricyclic antidepressants on self-stimulation in rats. In Cerletti, A., Bove, F.J. (eds.), *The Present Status of Psychotropic Drugs*. Amsterdam: Excerpta Medica, pp. 247–249.

Biggio, G., Casa, M., Corda, M., DiBello, C., Gessa, G.L. (1978) Stimulation of dopamine synthesis in caudate nucleus by intrastriatel enkephalins and antagonism by naloxone. *Science* 200:522–554.

Crow, T.J. (1970) Enhancement by cocaine of intracranial self-stimulation in the rat. *Life Sci.* 9:375–381.

Dole, V.P., Nyswander, M.E. (1967) Addiction—a metabolic disease. *Arch. Int. Med.* 120:19–24.

Esposito, R.U., Motola, A.H.D., Kornetsky, C. (1978) Cocaine: Acute effects on reinforcement thresholds for self-stimulation behavior to the medial forebrain bundle. *Pharmacol. Biochem. Behav.* 8:437–439.

Esposito, R.U., Perry, W., Kornetsky, C. (1980) Effects of d-amphetamine and naloxone on brain stimulation reward. *Psychopharmacol.* 69: 187–191.

Ettenberg, A., Pettit, H.O., Bloom, F.E., Koob, G.F. (1982) Heroin and cocaine intravenous self-administration in rats: mediation by separate neural systems. *Psychopharmacol.* 78:204–209.

Fibiger, H.C. (1978) Drugs and reinforcement mechanisms: a critical review of the catecholamine theory. *Ann. Rev. Pharmacol. Toxicol.* 18:37–56.

Gallistel, C.R., Shizgal, P., Yeomans, J.S. (1981) A portrait of the substrate for self-stimulation. *Psychol. Rev.* 88:228–273.

Glick, S.D., Cox, R.D. (1975) Dopaminergic and cholinergic influences on morphine self-administration in rats. *Res. Commun. Chem. Pathol. Pharmacol.* 12:17–24.

Gratton, A., Wise, R.A. (1985) Hypothalamic reward mechanisms: two first stage fiber populations with a cholinergic component. *Science* 227:545–548.

Hanson, H.M., Cimini-Venema, C.A. (1972) Effects of haloperidol on self-administration of morphine in rats. *Fed. Proc.* 31:503.

Holtzman, S.G. (1976) Comparison of the effects of morphine, pentazocine, cyclazocine, and amphetamine on intracranial self-stimulation in the rat. *Psychopharmacol.* 46:223–227.

Hubner, C., Kornetsky, C. (1984) The effects of heroin on brain-stimulation reward. *Soc. Neurosci. Absts.* 10:1106.

Hubner, C.B., Bain, G.T., Kornetsky, C. (1983) Morphine and d-amphetamine: effects on brain-stimulation reward. *Soc. Neurosci Abst.* 9:893.

Jaffe, J.H. (1984) Evaluating drug abuse treatment: a comment on the state of the art. In Tims, F.M., Ludford, J.P. (eds.), *Drug abuse treatment evaluation: strategies, progress, and prospects.* National Institute on Drug Abuse Research Monograph No. 51, DHHS pub. no. (ADM) 84–1329. Washington, D.C.: U.S. Government Printing Office, pp. 13–28.

Jasinski, D.R., Boren, J.J., Henningfield, J.E., Johnson, R.E., Lange, W.R., Lukas, S.E. (1983) Progress report from the NIDA Addiction Research Centers, Baltimore, Maryland. In Harris, L.S. (ed.), *Problems of drug dependence 1983.* National Institute on Drug

Abuse Research Monograph No. 49, DHHS pub. no. (ADM) 84-1316. Washington, D.C.: U.S. Government Printing Office, pp. 69–76.

Jasinski, D.R., Nutt, J.G. (1972) Progress report on the assessment program on the NIMH Addiction Center. In *Report of the thirty-fourth annual scientific meeting committee on problems of drug dependence.* Michigan: NIMH, pp. 442–477.

Khantzian, E.J. (1980) An ego/self theory of substance dependence. In Lettieri, D.J., Sayers, M., Pearson, H.W. (eds.), *Theories on drug abuse.* NIDA Research Monograph No. 30. Washington, D.C.: U.S. Government Printing Office, pp. 29–33.

Killam, K.F., Olds, J., Sinclair, J. (1957) Further studies on the effects of centrally acting drugs on self-stimulation. *J. Pharmacol. Exper. Ther.* 119:157.

Kornetsky, C., Bain, G. (1983) Effects of opiates on rewarding brain stimulation. In Smith, J.E., Lane, J.D. (eds.), *The Neurobiology of Opiate Reward Processes.* New York: Elsevier, pp. 237–256.

Kornetsky, C., Esposito, R.U., McLean, S., Jacobson, J.O. (1979) Intracranial self-stimulation thresholds: A model for the hedonic effects of drugs of abuse. *Arch. Gen. Psychiat.* 36: 289–292.

Kornetsky, C., Wheeling, H.S. (1982) An animal model for opiate induced euphoria and analgesia. *Ther Umsh/Revue Therapetique* 39:617–623.

Lorens, S.A., Sainati, S.M. (1978) Naloxone blocks the excitatory effect of ethanol and chlordiazepoxide on lateral hypothalamic self-stimulation behavior. *Life Sci.* 23:1359–1364.

Marcus, R., Kornetsky, C. (1974) Negative and positive intracranial reinforcement thresholds: effects of morphine. *Psychopharmacol.* 38: 1–13.

Olds, J., Killam, K.F., Bach-y-Rita, P. (1956) Self-stimulation of the brain used as a screening method for tranquilizing drugs. *Science* 124:265–266.

Olds, J., Milner, P. (1954) Positive reinforcement produced by electrical stimulation of septal area and other regions of rat brain. *J. Comp. Physiol. Psychol.* 47:419–427.

Olds, J., Travis, R.P. (1960) Effects of chlorpromazine, meprobamate, pentobarbital and morphine on self-stimulation. *J. Pharmacol. Exp. Ther.* 128:397–404.

Olds, M.E., Domino, E.F. (1969a) Comparison of muscarinic and nicotinic cholinergic agonists on self-stimulation behavior. *J. Pharmacol. Exp. Ther.* 166:189–204.

Olds, M.E., Domino, E.F. (1969b) Differential effects of cholinergic agonists on self-stimulation and escape behavior. *J. Pharmacol. Exp. Ther.* 170:157–167.

78 | Cocaine

Olds, M.E., Forbes, J.L. (1981) The central basis of motivation: Intracranial self-stimulation studies. *Ann. Rev. Psychol.* 32:523–574.

Overton, D.A. (1964) State-dependent or "dissociated" learning produced with pentobarbital. *J. Comp. Physiol. Psychol.* 57:3–12.

Perry, W., Esposito, R.U., Kornetsky, C. (1981) Effects of chronic naloxone treatment on brain-stimulation reward. *Pharmacol. Biochem. Behav.* 14:247–249.

Pettit, H.O., Ettenberg, A., Bloom, F.L., Koob, G.F. (1984) Destruction of dopamine in nucleus accumbens selectively attenuates cocaine but not heroin self-administration in rats. *Psychopharmacol.* 84:167–173.

Pollard, H., Lloren-Cortes, C., Schwartz, J.C. (1977a) Enkephalin receptors on dopaminergic neurons in rat striatum. *Nature* (Lond.) 268:745–747.

Pollard, H., Llorens, C., Bonnet, J.J., Coslentin, J., Schwartz, J.C. (1977b) Opiate receptors on mesolimbic dopaminergic neurons. *Neurosci. Lett.* 7:295–299.

Pozuelo, J., Kerr, F.W.L. (1972) Suppression of craving and other signs of dependence in morphine-addicted monkeys by administration of alpha-methyl-para-tyrosine. *Mayo Clin. Proc.* 47:621–628.

Prado-Alcala, R., Streather, A., Wise, R.A. (1984) Brain stimulation reward and dopamine terminal fields. II. Septal and cortical projections. *Brain Res.* 301:209–219.

Prado-Alcala, R., Wise, R.A. (1984) Brain stimulation reward and dopamine terminal fields. I. Caudate-putamen, nucleus accumbens and amygdala. *Brain Res.* 297:265–273.

Schaeffer, G.J., Michael, R.P. (1981) Threshold differences for naloxone and naltrexone in the hypothalamus and midbrain using fixed ratio brain self-stimulation in rats. *Psychopharmacol.* 74:17–22.

Schwartz, J.C., Pollard, H., Llorens, C., Malfroy, B., Gros, C., Pradelles, P., Dray, F. (1978) Endorphins and endorphin receptors in striatum: relationships with dopaminergic neurons. *Adv. Biochem. Psychopharmacol.* 18:245–264.

Seeger, T.F., Porrino, L.R., Esposito, R.U., Crane, A.M., Sullivan, T.L., Pert, A. (1984) Amphetamine effects on intracranial self-stimulation as assessed by the quantitative 2-deoxy-glucose method. *Soc. Neurosci. Abst.* 10:307.

Smith, J.E., Co. C., Freeman, M.E., Sands, M.P., Lane, J.D. (1980) Neurotransmitter turnover in rat striatum is correlated with morphine self-administration. *Nature* 287:152–154.

Sokoloff, L. (1982) The radioactive deoxyglucose method: theory, procedure and application for the assessment of local glucose utilization in the central nervous system. In Agranoff, B.W., and Aperson, M.H. (eds.), *Advances in Neurochemistry*. New York: Plenum, pp. 1–82.

Stapleton, J.M., Merriman, V.J., Coogle, C.L., Gelbard, S.D., Reid, L.D. (1979) Naloxone reduces pressing for intracranial stimulation of sites in the periaqueductal gray area, accumbens nucleus, substantia nigra, and lateral hypothalamus. *Physiol. Psychol.* 7:427–436.

Stark, P., Turk, J.A., Redman, C.E., Henderson, J.K. (1969) Sensitivity and specificity of positive reinforcing areas to neurosedatives, antidepressants, and stimulants. *J. Pharmacol. Exp. Ther.* 166: 163–169.

Stein, L. (1962) Effects of interactions of imipramine, chlorpromazine, reserpine, and amphetamine on self-stimulation: possible neurophysiological basis of depression. In Heath, R. (ed.), *Recent Advances in Biological Psychiatry*. New York: Plenum, pp. 288–309.

Stein, L. (1964) Self-stimulation of the brain and the central stimulant action of amphetamine. *Fed. Proc.* 23:836–850.

Stein, L., Ray, O.S. (1960) Brain stimulation reward "thresholds" self determined in the rat. *Psychopharmacol.* 1:251–856.

Unterwald, E.M., Kornetsky, C. (1984) Effects of concomitant pentazocine and tripelennamine on brain-stimulation reward. *Pharmacol. Biochem. Behav.* 21:961–964.

Unterwald, E.M., Kucharski, L.T., Williams, J.E.G., Kornetsky, C. (1984a) Tripelennamine: enhancement of brain-stimulation reward. *Life Sci.* 34:149–153.

Unterwald, E.M., Clark, J.A., Bain, G., Kornetsky, C. (1984b) The effects of ethanol on rewarding intracranial stimulation: rate and threshold measure. *Soc. Neurosci. Abst.* 10:572.

van der Kooy, D., LePiane, F.G., Phillips, A.G. (1977) Apparent independence of opiate reinforcement and electrical self-stimulation systems in rat brain. *Life Sci.* 20:981–986.

Wauquier, A., Niemegeers, C.J.E., Lal, H. (1974) Differential antagonism by naloxone of inhibitory effects of haloperidol and morphine on brain self-stimulation. *Psychopharmacol.* 37:303–310.

Weeks, J. (1962) Experimental morphine addiction: method for automatic intravenous injections in unrestrained rats. *Science* 138:143–144.

Wise, R.A., Bozarth, M.A. (1982) Action of drugs of abuse on brain reward systems: an update with specific attention to opiates. *Pharmacol. Biochem. Behav.* 17:239–243.

Wood, P.L., Stotland, M., Richard, J.W., Rackham, A. (1980) Actions of mu, kappa, sigma, delta and agonist/antagonist opiates on striatal dopaminergic function. *J. Pharmacol. Exp. Ther.* 215:697–703.

4 | Neural Substrates for Cocaine and Opiate Reinforcement

GEORGE F. KOOB, FRANCO J. VACCARINO,
MARIANNE AMALRIC, and NEAL R. SWERDLOW

DRUGS such as the psychomotor stimulants and opiates act like other natural reinforcers that increase the probability of a response: they strengthen and maintain operant behavior, for example, drug self-administration (Pickens & Harris, 1968; Woods & Schuster, 1968; Deneau et al., 1969; Thompson & Pickens, 1970; Yokel & Pickens, 1973; Schuster & Thompson, 1969). Given the neuro-pharmacological advances that allow for relatively specific inactivation of specific neurochemical systems, it becomes feasible to examine the neurobiological mechanisms for these reinforcing effects. Such studies would not only provide information on the basic mechanisms of action for the behavioral effects of these drugs, but also may shed insight into the neurobiological organization of reinforcement processes themselves.

In stimulant and opiate self-administration, animals maintain a relatively stable level of drug intake over time with very regular interinjection intervals, particularly with short daily sessions (approximately 3 hours) (Ettenberg et al., 1982; Koob et al., 1984). In response to changes in this injection dose, animals typically show an inverse relationship between dose and number of injections per session—low doses produce a higher number of self-injections than higher doses (see Fig. 4.1). More important for the present context is the nature of the change in behavior following treatment with a pharmacological antagonist. Treatment with the opiate receptor antagonist produces an increase in the number of self-injections of morphine (Goldberg et al., 1971; Weeks & Collins, 1976; Ettenberg et al., 1982). This increase is generally considered to reflect a

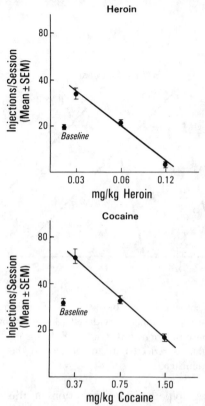

FIGURE 4.1. Dose-response relationships for cocaine (top) and heroin (bottom) self-administration in rats. Rats were allowed daily 3-hour access to cocaine (0.75 mg/kg/injection) or heroin (0.06 mg/kg/injection) on a continuous reinforcement schedule. After baseline stable responding (± 20% mean for 3 days) was established, rats were subjected to a doubling of the dose followed by a return to baseline followed by a halving of the dose on 3 successive test days. Results are expressed as mean ± S.E.M., for cocaine $n = 6$; for heroin $n = 4$.

competitive functional interaction; the rat presumably increases its drug self-administration to compensate for the decreased effectiveness of morphine as a reinforcer in the presence of partial receptor occupancy by the antagonist. Consequently, an increase in self-administration resulting from administration of an opiate antagonist is qualitatively similar to the effects of decreasing the dose of drug

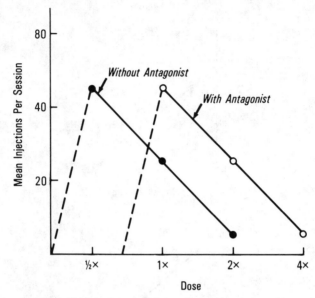

FIGURE 4.2. Hypothetical model of the effects of a pharmacological antagonist on the dose-response function with self-administration. Note the shift of the dose-response function to the right. With this model, a decrease in reinforcement value is reflected in an increase in the number of drug injections self-administered.

per injection. A hypothetical description of this relationship is shown in Figure 4.2.

Catecholamines have been strongly implicated in the reinforcing properties of psychomotor stimulants (Pickens et al., 1978). More specifically, the reinforcing properties of psychomotor stimulants have been linked to the activation of central dopamine (DA) neurons and their post-synaptic receptors. When the synthesis of catecholamines is inhibited by administering alpha-methyl-para-tyrosine, an attenuation of the reinforcing effects of psychomotor stimulants occurs (Pickens et al., 1968; Jonsson et al., 1971). Furthermore, low doses of DA antagonists will increase the response rates for intravenous injections of d-amphetamine (Davis & Smith, 1975; Yokel & Wise, 1975,1976). These authors hypothesized that a partial blockade of DA receptors produced a partial blockade of the reinforcing effects of d-amphetamine. Thus, animals are thought to compensate for decreases in the magnitude of the reinforcer by

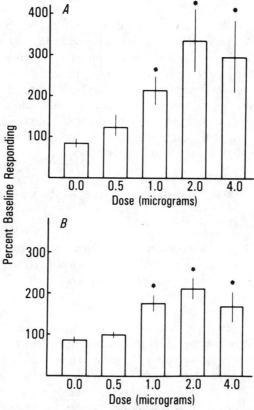

FIGURE 4.3. The effects of i.c.v. MN treatment on responding for heroin over the first hour (*A*) and over the total 3-hour self-administration session (*B*). Response rates were expressed as the percentage of baseline responding. Asterisks indicate that the treatment dose was significantly different from the saline treatment, $p<0.05$, Newman-Keuls test. Six rats were tested across all drug treatments. The day prior to i.c.v. injections was used as the baseline day. (Taken with permission from Vaccarino, Pettit, Bloom & Koob, 1985).

increasing their self-administration behavior (see above and Fig. 4.3). The role of dopamine in the reinforcing properties of cocaine was extended by the observation that 6-hydroxydopamine lesions of the nucleus accumbens produce extinction-like responding and a significant and long-lasting reduction in self-administration of cocaine over days (Roberts et al., 1977, 1980; Lyness, Friedle & Moore, 1979).

These results demonstrated that postsynaptic blockade of dopamine receptors or destruction of presynaptic dopamine terminals in the region of the nucleus accumbens significantly decreased the reinforcing value of psychomotor stimulants. Unknown was how these results extended to other self-administered drugs and more specifically to opiates. Although animals will readily self-administer opiates and even self-administer opioid peptides directly into the brain, the opiate receptors critical for systemic opiate self-administration were largely unexplored.

NEUROCHEMICAL SUBSTRATES OF HEROIN REINFORCEMENT

The Role of Peripheral Opiate Receptors

In humans, opiate injection is accompanied by "a warm flushing of the skin and sensations in the lower abdomen described by addicts as similar in intensity and quality to sexual orgasm" (Jaffe, 1980; for earlier reference see Wikler, 1952). Known as the "rush," this sensation lasts for approximately 45 sec and is generally thought to be one of the motivating factors involved in opiate use (Jaffe, 1980). However, it is not clear that this rush is mediated by direct drug action on the central nervous system, since it is well established that interoceptive autonomic stimuli have an important role in the maintenance of heroin consumption in humans (Meyer & Mirin, 1979). More operationally, it is not known whether the reinforcing properties of opiates that result from the sensations associated with this rush arise directly from activation of opiate receptors in the central nervous system or from opiate receptors localized in the periphery.

We compared the potency and efficacy of naloxone and naltrexone with their quaternary derivatives in antagonizing the reinforcing properties of heroin. The quaternary derivatives of naloxone and naltrexone were chosen because of their potentially selective antagonist action that excludes them from penetrating through the blood brain barrier. As a result, they can antagonize opiate effects on peripheral opiate receptors as inferred from their ability to antagonize morphine effects on gastrointenstinal transit, but do not antagonize central opiate actions on pain (Tavani et al., 1979). Recent studies have confirmed conditionally the peripheral selectivity of these compounds (Bianchi et al., 1982). Furthermore, others have reported that quaternary naltrexone was ineffective as an antagonist of the morphine discriminative stimulus or in precipitating abstinence in morphine-dependent rhesus monkeys (Valentino et al., 1981).

In rats self-administering heroin (0.06 mg/kg/injection in daily 5-hour sessions), low doses (0.05 to 0.2 mg/kg) of naloxone and naltrexone produced dose-dependent increases in self-administration; at higher doses (10 to 30 mg/kg) these drugs produced transient decreases in heroin self-administration followed by recovery (Ettenberg et al., 1982; Koob et al., 1984). The quaternary derivatives were ineffective as antagonists of heroin self-administration in doses 200X greater than the effective antagonist dose of naloxone or naltrexone (Koob et al., 1984). These results support the hypothesis that the acute reinforcing properties of i.v. opiates associated with the sensation of the "rush" involve opiate receptors located within the central nervous system and do not involve peripheral opiate receptors (see Koob et al., 1984).

In support of a selective peripheral action for these quaternary compounds, others have shown that the quaternary derivatives of opiate antagonists do not induce withdrawal signs in morphine-dependent dogs or monkeys at doses that blocked morphine-induced intestinal spike potentials (Russell et al., 1982). Also, the present results are unlikely to be explained simply on the basis of differential binding potency of the antagonists to opiate receptors. Naltrexone is only about 50 times more potent than quaternary naltrexone in an *in vitro* assay of opiate antagonist activity (Valentino et al., 1981). In our laboratories, MN is approximately one-tenth as potent as naloxone in displacing morphine from opiate receptor sites (Koob et al., unpublished results). In addition, others have shown *in vivo* that the dose (1 mg/kg) of naloxone methobromide required for complete antagonism of morphine (5 mg/kg) on gastrointestinal transport in rats was only 2 to 4 times higher than the dose of naloxone hydrochloride required to produce the same effect (Bianchi et al., 1982).

The Role of Brain Dopamine Receptors

Previous studies have shown that centrally acting opiate receptor antagonists increase heroin self-administration and centrally acting dopamine receptor antagonists increase cocaine self-administration.

It was not known whether these effects were pharmacologically independent of each other. To examine whether dopamine receptor antagonists alter the self-administration of opiates, rats trained to self-administer heroin (0.06 mg/kg/inj) intravenously for daily 3-hour sessions were subjected to a series of doses of the dopamine receptor antagonist, alpha-flupenthixol. Alpha-flupenthixol, in doses that dose-dependently increased cocaine self-administration, failed to increase heroin self-administration. Indeed, the only significant effect on heroin self-administration was a decrease in self-administration at 0.4 mg/kg of alpha-flupenthixol, a cataleptic dose. Naltrexone produced a dose-dependent increase in self-administration, but had no effect on cocaine self-administration (Ettenberg et al., 1982). These results confirmed those observed by others using other antagonists of opiates and dopamine (Goldberg, Woods & Schuster, 1971; Yokel & Wise, 1976; Weeks & Collins, 1976; DeWit & Wise, 1977).

The increased responding observed with the respective antagonist for each drug is thought to occur because the antagonist drugs presumably compete with the same synaptic sites as those influenced by the self-administered drug. Heroin, for example, is assumed to be converted to morphine in the brain and the morphine binds to central opiate receptors (Way & Adler, 1960). Cocaine is thought to enhance dopaminergic transmission by blocking the reuptake of presynaptic dopamine (Patrick, Synder & Barchas, 1975). Therefore, the net reinforcement produced by combining the self-administered drug and its specific antagonist is equivalent to the net effect on neurotransmission; animals respond to increasing doses of the antagonist by increasing the amount of drug self-administered. Of particular significance was the observation that low doses of alpha-flupenthixol did not increase responding for heroin, nor did naltrexone increase cocaine-reinforced responding. The specificity with which these antagonists exerted their behavioral effects strongly suggests that separate neural substrates are responsible for the reinforcing actions of heroin and cocaine (Ettenberg et al., 1982).

Location Within the CNS of the Opiate Receptors Critical for Heroin Reinforcement

The mesolimbic dopamine system has not only been accorded an important role in psychomotor stimulant reward; it has also been hypothesized that this system is critical for the reinforcing properties of opiates (Bozarth & Wise, 1981a). For example, rats will self-administer morphine into the ventral tegmental area (VTA) (Bozarth & Wise, 1981b), and more recent studies have shown that rats will directly self-administer D-ala^2-methionine enkephalin into the nucleus accumbens (Goeders, Lane & Smith, 1984). Indeed, Britt and Wise (1983) have shown that administration of quaternary nalorphine into the ventral tegmental area but not the nucleus accumbens attenuated the self-administration of heroin. Our next series of studies were designed to extend these observations by examining the effects of methyl naloxonium chloride, a naloxone derivative known not to cross the blood brain barrier on i.v. heroin self-administration after microinjection into the cerebral ventricles, the ventral tegmental area (VTA), or nucleus accumbens (N.Acc.).

Rats were implanted with intracerebral injections cannulas aimed above the lateral ventricle, the VTA, or N.Acc. They were trained to self-administer heroin (0.06 mg/kg/injection) intravenously. Following stable responding (3 days where baseline days were ± 20% of mean for the 3-day period) each rat received a bilateral microinjection of methylnaloxonium chloride (MN) into either the lateral ventricle, N.Acc. or VTA 10 minutes prior to self-administration tests. The following MN doses were tested: 0.0, 0.125, 0.25, 0.5, and 1.0 (2 µl volume over 2 minutes). Doses were administered in ascending order with a minimum of three "no-pretreatment days" separating drug tests.

The results showed that lateral ventricular injections of MN produced a dose dependent increase in heroin self-administration similar to that observed for systemic injections of naloxone (Fig. 4.3). Effective doses ranged from 1.0 to 4.0 µg (for details, see Vaccarino, Pettit, Bloom & Koob, 1985). Similar results were obtained following injections of MN into the VTA with no effect of MN until reaching a dose of 1.0 µg (Fig. 4.4). However, MN injected into the nucleus accumbens was approximately eightfold more potent at increasing self-administration of heroin. Significant increases were observed in doses as low as from 0.125 to 0.25 µg with peak effects at 0.5 µg (Fig. 4.5) (for details see Vaccarino, Bloom & Koob, 1985).

Following completion of MN testing, rats injected in the N.Acc. were switched from heroin to cocaine reward. Following stable responding on cocaine (0.75 mg/kg/injection), these rats received

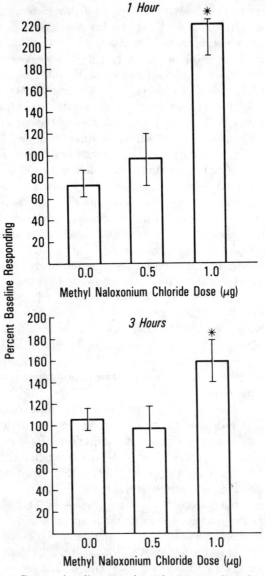

FIGURE 4.4. Percent baseline (pre-drug day) responding for i.v. heroin during the first hour (top graph) and for the total 3 hours (bottom graph) of the heroin self-administration session following MN injections into the ventral tegmental area. Asterisks indicate a significant difference ($p<.05$) from both saline vehicle (0.0 dose) and 0.5 μg MN, Duncan Multiple Range a posteriori test (taken with permission from Vaccarino, Bloom & Koob, 1985).

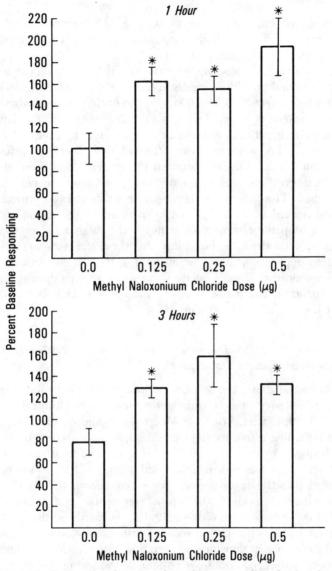

FIGURE 4.5. Percent baseline (pre-drug day) responding for i.v. heroin during the first hour (top graph) and for the total 3 hours (bottom graph) of the heroin self-administration session following MN injections into the nucleus accumbens. Asterisks indicate a significant difference ($p<.05$) from saline vehicle (0.0 dose, Duncan Multiple Range a posteriori test. (Taken with permission from Vaccarino, Bloom & Koob, 1985).

intra-N.Acc. microinjections of 0.5 µg MN (optimal dose) 10 minutes prior to the self-administration session. MN had no effect on cocaine self-administration.

These overall results suggest that the nucleus accumbens is an important and possibly critical substrate for the reinforcing actions of opiates. Effective doses of MN in the nucleus accumbens were approximately 8 times lower than those observed for lateral ventricular injections. Somewhat surprisingly, injections of MN into the VTA were no more effective than lateral ventricular injections. The difference between the present results and those reported previously using quarternary nalorphine are not easily explained. The present results suggest that the receptors critical for opiate reward may be localized on neurons in the region of the N.Acc. dopamine projection, namely, the mesolimbic dopamine system. To address the possibility that these receptors were localized on dopamine neurons terminating in the nucleus accumbens, subsequent work in our laboratory examined whether destruction of presynaptic dopamine terminals in the nucleus accumbens would alter heroin self-administration.

The Role of Presynaptic Dopamine Terminals in the Nucleus Accumbens on Opiate and Cocaine Reinforcement

As discussed above, the mesolimbic dopamine system appears to be critical for psychomotor stimulant reinforcement (Roberts et al., 1977, 1980; Lyness, Friedle & Moore, 1979) and thus any hypotheses regarding a role for dopamine in opioid reinforcement would likely focus on this same mesolimbic system. This is particularly relevant since rats will maintain self-administration of morphine applied directly into the brain region containing the mesolimbic dopamine cell bodies, the ventral tegmental area (Phillips & LePiane, 1980; Bozarth & Wise, 1981b). To clarify further the role of mesolimbic dopamine neurons in opiate reinforcement we examined the effects of dopamine denervation of the nucleus accumbens on both heroin and cocaine self-administration simultaneously.

Rats were trained to self-administer intravenously heroin (0.06 mg/kg/injection) and cocaine (0.75 mg/kg/injection) for 3 hours on alternate days. This alternate drug self-administration procedure was continued until stable intake and titration on both drugs had occurred. For each rat, each drug was delivered via a given lever (left or right), and a colored light (red or yellow) was used as a constant discriminative stimulus which was turned on at the onset of the infusion and remained on for 20 sec.

Animals that showed stable baselines over 3 days with each drug (i.e., those rats that varied less than 20% of the mean for any individual trial) were given an intracerebral injection of either 6-hydroxydopamine (6-OHDA) or vehicle into the nucleus accumbens, as described previously (Joyce & Koob, 1981). These lesions produced a 94% depletion of dopamine in the nucleus accumbens but no significant decrease in the anterior striatum (Pettit et al., 1984). Four days following the lesion the rats were allowed to resume the alternating schedule of self-administration described above. The 6-OHDA lesions initially produced an attenuation in both cocaine and heroin self-administration on the first self-administration trial post-lesion. Subsequently, heroin responding recovered with time gradually increasing to 76% of pre-lesion baseline levels on average. In contrast, cocaine responding continued to decrease over trials after 6-OHDA. By the fifth trial post-lesion, cocaine self-administration rates were reduced to 30% of pre-lesion baseline levels and this percent change was significantly different from that for heroin rates (see Pettit et al., 1984). No significant differences in responding to cocaine or heroin post-lesion were seen in sham operated rats (Pettit et al., 1984). However, there was a significant increase in responding over time for both drugs.

To eliminate the possibility that the group differences in baseline rates of responding for post-lesion heroin and cocaine could explain the treatment effects, individual response records were examined for those animals displaying approximately equal pre-lesion response rates for cocaine and heroin infusions. In three such animals, heroin responses were distinctly higher than cocaine responses post-lesion, demonstrating an absolute as well as relative difference in responding (for details, see Pettit et al., 1984). These results demonstrate that selective lesions of the presynaptic dopamine input to the nucleus accumbens can significantly attenuate cocaine self-administration without influencing heroin responding.

An important factor in this study was that the effects of each lesion could be measured on the two independent drug variables almost simultaneously. Thus, differential effects could not be attributed to nonsimilar DA depletion levels, since for each subject the lesion had specific effects on the self-administration of cocaine and heroin that were compared within individuals to pre-lesion rates. Thus, these results have direct implications as to the neural substrates responsible for the reinforcing properties of both psychomotor stimulants and opioids, and suggest that the reinforcing properties of heroin are at some point independent of the dopaminergic neural systems mediating the reinforcing properties of cocaine.

NEUROCHEMICAL SUBSTRATES OF HEROIN ACTIVATION

Role of Brain Dopamine Receptors

As discussed above, opiates or opioid peptides injected directly into the region of the N.Acc or the VTA produce motor activation. The activation produced by VTA injection can be reversed by destruction of presynaptic dopamine terminals in the nucleus accumbens (Kelley et al., 1980; Stinus et al., 1980). However, a recent study has provided evidence for the presence of a DA-independent substrate of opioid-induced locomotor activation (Kalivas et al., 1983). Here microinjections of DALA into the N.Acc produced locomotor activation that was not attenuated by destruction of the mesolimbic DA system (Kalivas et al., 1983). Also, intra-VTA DALA injections produced an increased DOPAC/DA ratio while intra-N.Acc DALA injections had no such effect (Kalivas et al., 1983). Based on these findings, the authors suggested that while activation of opiate receptors in the VTA appears to produce a DA-dependent locomtor activation, activation of opiate receptors in the N.Acc produces a DA-independent locomotor activation (Kalivas et al., 1983).

The present experiment was designed to investigate the role of the mesolimbic DA system in the expression of locomotor activation induced by systemic heroin administration. To this end, the effects of systemic neuroleptic treatment on heroin and amphetamine-induced locomotor activation were investigated.

To measure the locomotor response to heroin and amphetamine, the rats were first pre-exposed to the photocell cages for 3 hours at least 2 days prior to a test day to overcome the potential stressful nature of a novel environment. On the test day, rats were pretreated with one of the following doses of alpha-flupenthixol: 0, 0.05, 0.1, and 0.2 mg/kg 1.0 hour before being placed in the photocell cages.

The rats were then placed in the photocell cages for a habituation period of 1.5 hours, after which they were injected with either *d*-amphetamine (0.35 mg/kg) s.c. or heroin (0.5 mg/kg) s.c. and monitored for another 3 hours.

Heroin, injected subcutaneously at a dose of 0.5 mg/kg, produced an initial catatonic-like state lasting 10 to 30 minutes, which was followed by a period of increased locomotor activation that lasted approximately 90 to 120 minutes. The increased locomotor activation reached a peak at about 90 minutes after the heroin injection (Fig. 4.6). Alpha-flupenthixol had little effect on heroin locomotion at the lower doses but produced an attenuation at the 0.2 mg/kg dose (Fig. 4.6).

The rats receiving amphetamine showed the characteristic immediate increase in locomotion which lasted for approximately 40 to 60 minutes. However, alpha-flupenthixol attenuated amphetamine locomotion at all three doses (0.05, 0.1, and 0.2 mg/kg) (Fig. 4.6).

The results show that alpha-flupenthixol, a DA antagonist, blocked amphetamine-induced locomotion at all three doses tested. This finding is consistent with numerous other studies indicating that amphetamine-induced locomotion is dependent on DA function (Joyce & Koob, 1981; Kelly et al., 1975; Koob et al., 1981). In contrast to amphetamine, heroin-induced locomotion was significantly affected by alpha-flupenthixol, except at the highest dose tested (0.2 mg/kg). The fact that alpha-flupenthixol had no effect on heroin locomotion at doses that blocked amphetamine locomotion (0.05 and 0.1 mg/kg) suggests that DA systems do not play a primary role in the expression of heroin-induced locomotion.

Location Within the CNS of the Opiate Receptors Critical for Heroin-Induced Motor Activation

At low doses, systemic administration of opiates in rats produces analgesia and locomotor activation; at higher doses, a state of immobility is followed by an increase in locomotor activity (Babbini & Davis, 1972). The locomotor activation observed in rats following systemic opiate treatment can be reproduced by intraventricular injections of endorphins and is believed to be a reflection of the mood-altering properties of opiates (Koob & Bloom, 1983). A number of studies have been directed at identifying the central

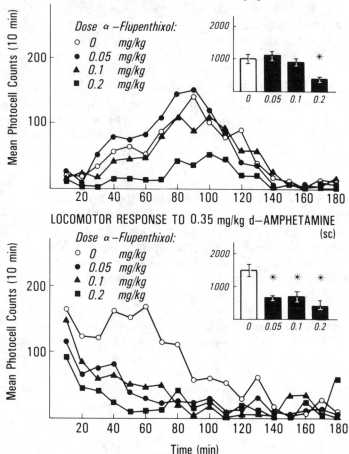

FIGURE 4.6. *Top:* Effects of alpha-flupenthixol on the locomotor response after s.c. injection of heroin (0.5 mg/kg). Rats were pretreated with alpha-flupenthixol and, 60 minutes later, habituated to the photocell cages. Ninety minutes later the rats were injected with heroin. *Bottom:* Effects of alpha-flupenthixol on the locomotor response after s.c. injection of amphetamine (0.35 mg/kg). Rats were pretreated and tested as in the top graph. Asterisks indicate a significant difference from saline, $p < .05$, Duncan Multiple Range a posteriori test. Inserts show the mean total counts for 180 min ± S.E.M. The present data is based on an independent group design. $N = 8$ in each group. (Taken with permission from Vaccarino et al., 1986)

substrates for opiate-induced locomotor activation. These studies have depended primarily on intracerebral injection techniques in which the locomotor response to direct intracerebral injections of opiates or opioid peptides was measured (Broekkamp et al., 1979; Bloom et al., 1976; Joyce & Iversen, 1979; Pert & Sivit, 1977; Stinus et al., 1980). Results from these studies have suggested that the mesolimbic dopamine (DA) system is critical for the expression of opiate-induced locomotor activation. For example, microinjections of morphine or opioid peptides into the ventral tegmental area (VTA), source of the mesolimbic DA cell bodies, produced an increase in locomotor activity which resembles that observed following systemic stimulant treatment (Broekkamp et al., 1979; Kelley et al., 1980; Stinus et al., 1980). Also, 6-OHDA lesions of the mesolimbic DA system or microinjections of DA receptor antagonists block the locomotor activation induced by intra-VTA microinjections of opiates (Kelley et al., 1980; Stinus et al., 1980).

However, other authors have focused on the role of the nucleus accumbens because it is a brain structure containing a relatively high concentration of opiate receptors (Pert & Sivit, 1977; Kalivas et al., 1983; Bunney, Massari & Pert, 1984). These workers have shown that direct administration of morphine or d-alanine methionine enhephalin into the nucleus accumbens produces an increase in locomotor activity. The locomotor stimulant effects of morphine were antagonized by systemic injections of naloxone but not by haloperidol, a dopaminergic antagonist (Pert & Sivit, 1977). In addition, 6-hydroxydopamine-induced destruction of the DA terminals in the nucleus accumbens failed to block the locomotor activating effect of opioid peptides; in fact, this treatment appears to produce a "cross-supersensitivity" (Kalivas et al., 1983), making rats unresponsive to cocaine but more responsive to opioids.

The present series of experiments were designed to examine the role of the opiate receptors in the mesolimbic dopamine system in systemic opiate-induced locomotor activation. Locomotor activation was induced by injecting a low dose of heroin (0.5 mg/kg) subcutaneously and measuring motor activity in photocell cages. An attempt was made to block this activation by injecting methylnaloxonium intracerebroventricularly or intracerebrally into the nucleus accumbens or ventral tegmental area.

Heroin injected subcutaneously at a dose of 0.5 mg/kg elicited a biphasic locomotor response. An initial cataleptic phase (10 to 30

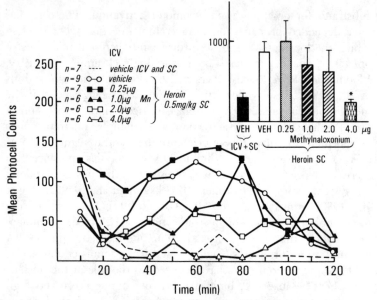

FIGURE 4.7. Mean photocell counts for 2 hours following intraventricular injection of saline or MN at different doses (0.25, 1.0, 2.0, 4.0 mg) and 1 minute later, subcutaneous injection of heroin (0.5 mg/kg). Insert: Locomotor activity counts for the total 120 min. Asterisk indicates significant difference from control (heroin s.c., vehicle i.c.v.) $p < 0.05$ by Student's t-test, following overall significant ANOVA; see text. (Taken with permission from Amalric and Koob, 1985)

min) was followed by a long-lasting period (40 to 120 min) of enhanced locomotor activity interrupted by bursts of stereotyped behavior (gnawing, licking, etc.). The activity reached a peak around 1 hour after injection time and lasted up to 2 hours (see Fig. 4.7).

The intracerebroventricular injection of methylnaloxonium (MN) at doses ranging from 1 μg to 4 μg decreased the locomotor activity for the two hours following the injection, in a dose-dependent way (see Fig. 4.7). Lateral ventricular injections did not significantly reverse the initial depressant effects of heroin (0 to 30 min), but the highest dose of 4 μg did reverse the subsequent hyperactivity (for details, see Amalric & Koob, 1985).

After MN injection into the VTA, locomotor activity was not significantly higher than the control group (heroin alone) during the

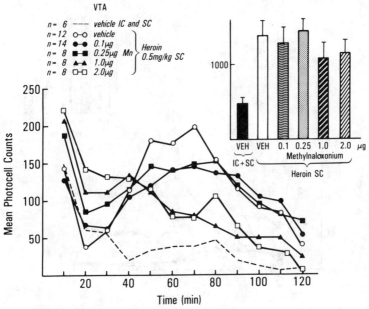

FIGURE 4.8. Locomotor responses for 2 hours following bilateral VTA infusion of methylnaloxonium (0.1, 0.25, 1.0, 2.0 μg total dose) followed 1 minute later by a subcutaneous injection of heroin (0.5 mg/kg). Insert: Total photocell counts for the 2 hours. (Taken with permission from Amalric and Koob, 1985)

first 30 minutes. However, some depression of the activity was observed during 2 hours at the highest doses (1.0 and 2.0 μg); see Figure 4.8. After MN injection into the nucleus accumbens, doses (1.0 and 2.0 μg) that induced only an attenuation of locomotor activity when injected into the VTA completely blocked by heroin-induced activation throughout all of the testing period when injected into the N.Acc (Fig. 4.9). Also, the lowest dose of MN (0.1 μg total dose) resulted in a significant general activation in the first 30 min depressant phase, similar to the tendency observed for 0.25 μg injected into the ventricle. A dose as low as 0.25 μg MN significantly reversed the subsequent hyperactivity (40 to 120 min) (for details, see Amalric & Koob, 1985). These data suggest that both the N.Acc. and VTA mediate some aspects of heroin-induced motor activation in rats but possibly via different neurochemical mechanisms.

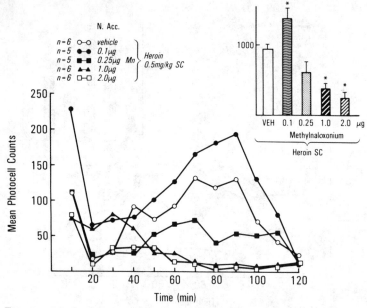

FIGURE 4.9. Locomotor response for 2 hours following bilateral N.Acc.-infusion of methylnaloxonium (0.1, 0.25, 1.0, 2.0 µg total) followed by a subcutaneous injection of heroin (0.5 mg/kg). Insert: total photocell counts for the 2 hours. Asterisks indicate significant difference from control, $p < 0.05$ by Student's t-test, following overall significant ANOVA. (Taken with permission from Amalric and Koob, 1985)

For example, intracerebral injection of opiates or opioid peptides into the ventral tegmental area results in an increase of locomotor activity and a general behavioral activation (Joyce & Iversen, 1979; Kelley et al., 1980; Stinus et al., 1980). This VTA activation is likely to be due to an increased release of DA in the mesolimbic areas, since the VTA response to d-alanine, d-leucine enhephaline was antagonized by a dopaminergic receptor antagonist (alpha-flupenthixol) (Joyce et al., 1981), or by destruction of the mesolimbic DA system, with 6-OHDA (Kelley et al., 1980; Stinus et al., 1980).

However, Pert and Sivit (1977) also have reported that microinjections of morphine into the nucleus accumbens resulted in an increase in spontaneous motor activity in rats. A significant elevation in locomotion and rearing preceded by a cataleptic phase, depending on the dose injected, was also seen after d-alanine methionine enkephalin microinjection into the N.Acc (Havemann et al., 1983; Kalivas et al., 1983; Pert & Sivit, 1977). In contrast to the activation following opiate injected into the VTA, this effect is not antagonized by haloperidol (a dopaminergic antagonist) (Pert & Sivit, 1977), nor by 6-OHDA depletion of DA in the accumbens (Kalivas et al., 1983), suggesting that opiates can increase motility in this region by a nondopaminergic action.

However, an important involvement of the N.Acc. in the opiate-induced activation is suggested by our results. The blockade of heroin-induced activation is more dramatic when MN is injected into the N.Acc. Furthermore, lower doses are required in the N.Acc. to attenuate the locomotor stimulation, significantly lower than those required to block motor activation via the intracerebroventricular route.

Role of Presynaptic Dopamine Terminals in the Nucleus Accumbens on Heroin-Induced Motor Activation

The present experiment was designed to test the hypothesis that the opiate receptors in the region of the nucleus accumbens responsible for the blockade heroin-induced locomotion are located on presynaptic dopaminergic fibers. The results where dopaminergic receptor blockade failed to block heroin locomotion except at high doses (Figure 4.6) argues against this hypothesis, but a more direct, test would be to remove the mesolimbic dopaminergic input and examine whether this manipulation would alter heroin-induced locomotion. Based on the results above, it was hypothesized that destruction of mesolimbic DA fibers, which are known to be critical for the expression of amphetamine locomotion (Kelly et al., 1973), should result in a blockade of amphetamine locomotion but have little effect on heroin locomotion.

Two groups of eight rats each were subjected to either 6-OHDA lesions of the N.Acc. (lesion group) or vehicle injection into the N.Acc. (sham group) as described earlier. Eight days following surgery rats were first pre-exposed to the photocell cages for 3 hours to habituate the rats to the novel environment. The following day rats were placed in the photocell cages for a habituation period of 1.5 hours, after which they were injected with heroin (0.5 mg/kg) s.c.

and monitored for an additional 3 hours. Seventy-two hours later animals were tested for their locomotor response to d-amphetamine (0.35 mg/kg) s.c., using the same procedure. As described previously, heroin injected subcutaneously at a dose of 0.5 mg/kg produced an initial catatonic phase (10 to 30 min) which was followed by a period of increased locomotor activation lasting approximately 90 to 120 minutes. As can be seen in Figure 4.10 (top graph, sham group), the increased locomotor activation reached a peak at about 90 minutes after the heroin injection. There was no significant change in locomotion produced by heroin in the lesion group (see Fig. 4.10). However, as predicted, the 6-OHDA lesion of the N.Acc. significantly attenuated amphetamine-induced locomotion (see Fig. 4.10).

These results showing that destruction of dopamine terminals in the N.Acc. significantly attenuate amphetamine but not heroin locomotion indicate that mesolimbic dopamine fibers are not essential for the expression of opiate-induced locomotion. This observation combined with the results showing resistance of heroin locomotion to dopamine receptor blockade suggests that the activation produced by systemic opiates, as with the reinforcing property of systemic opiates, is independent of a critical dopaminergic link. In addition, the observation that the locomotor-activating properties of systemic heroin can be blocked by injections of low doses of methylnaloxonium chloride into the N.Acc. suggests that the opiate receptors critical for this effect are located postsynaptic to the dopamine terminals.

HYPOTHETICAL NEUROPHARMACOLOGICAL MODEL FOR REINFORCING AND ACTIVATING PROPERTIES OF COCAINE AND OPIATES

To summarize our results, rats that intravenously self-administered cocaine increased their responding rates when pretreated with the DA antagonist alpha-flupenthixol; this was interpreted as a decrease in the reinforcing value of cocaine. These rats did not exhibit a similar compensatory increase in responding when pretreated with the opiate antagonist, naltrexone. However, rats that intravenously self-administered *heroin* did show a compensatory increase in responding after systemic naloxone, or after microinjection of

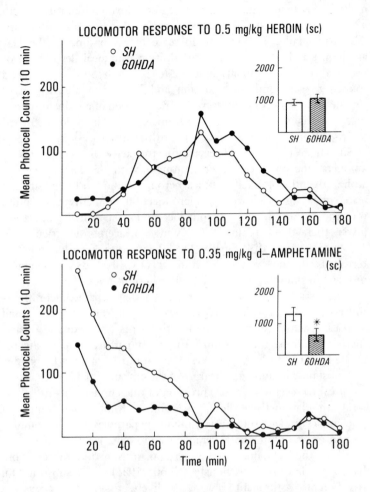

FIGURE 4.10. *Top:* Effects of 6-OHDA lesions of the N.Acc. on the locomotor response after s.c. injection of heroin (0.5 mg/kg). Rats were habituated to the photocell cages for 90 minutes after which they were injected with heroin. *Bottom:* Effects of 6-OHDA lesions of the N.Acc. on the locomotor response after s.c. injection of amphetamine (0.35 mg/kg). Rats were tested as in the top graph. Asterisk indicates a difference from sham lesion group, $p<0.05$, main effect ANOVA. Inserts show the mean total counts for 180 min ± S.E.M. for 8 rats in the sham and lesion group, respectively.

101

methylnaloxonium (quaternary analog of naloxone) into the N.Acc. This was interpreted as a decrease in the reinforcing value of heroin. These rats failed to show an increase in responding to the DA antagonist alpha-flupenthixol. In addition, the local destruction of presynaptic DA terminals in the N.Acc. with 6-OHDA in rats trained to self-administer cocaine and heroin on alternate days revealed a time-dependent decrease or extinction of cocaine responding, whereas in these same rats heroin self-administration returned to 76% of pre-lesion baseline by the 5th trial post-lesion.

Similar results were observed for the activating properties of amphetamine and heroin. Pretreatment with the DA antagonist alpha-flupenthixol failed to block heroin locomotion except at high (cataleptic) doses. However, microinjection of methylnaloxonium into the N.Acc. blocked heroin locomotion at doses significantly lower than those required following intracerebroventricular or VTA injection of MN. Finally, local destruction of presynaptic DA terminals in the N.Acc. with 6-OHDA blocked amphetamine induced locomotion but failed to alter heroin-induced activity.

These results support the hypothesis that separate neurotransmitter-specific pathways are responsible for the reinforcing and activating actions of psychomotor stimulants (cocaine) and opiates (heroin) and raise the possibility that these pathways may converge at the level of the N.Acc. Other work in our laboratory has shown the substantia innominata (a target of the output of the N.Acc.) to be a critical connection in the expression of nucleus accumbens behavioral stimulation (Swerdlow, Swanson & Koob, 1984), and this nucleus accumbens-substantia innominata pathway may be common second-order link for both stimulant and opiate reinforcement.

A hypothetical model for these drug neurotransmitter interactions has been described previously (Koob, 1986). The substrate for psychomotor stimulant reward is likely to be the *presynaptic* dopamine terminals located in the nucleus accumbens that originate in the ventral tegmental area. However, an important substrate for heroin reward is most likely to *postsynaptic* to this dopamine system but probably also located in the region of the nucleus accumbens. Hypothetically, heroin (which is converted to morphine in the brain) would act by directly mimicing some endogenous opioid peptide at opiate receptors in the nucleus accumbens. Which opioid peptides are involved and from where the cell bodies for these peptides derive are questions for future work.

In addition, these studies provide evidence to show that in the rat the neural/neurochemical substrates for processing the reinforcing and stimulant properties of psychomotor stimulants and opiates may be similar, if not identical. Parallel manipulations using dopamine receptor antagonists and 6-OHDA lesions produce parallel results. How far this parallelism continues in further processing is under current investigation. However, this overlap brings additional impetus to earlier hypotheses relating reinforcement and motor function (see Glickman & Schiff, 1967).

Of perhaps more general interest, our results speak to the question of multiple versus single critical substrates for reinforcement in the brain. For example, the above studies show independent neurochemical substrates for cocaine and heroin reinforcement and undermine hypotheses suggesting that dopamine systems are a critical substrate for all reinforcement. Clearly, opiate reinforcement can occur independent of activation of the mesolimbic dopamine system. However, these results do point to an important role for the region of the nucleus accumbens and its connections in the neurobiological mechanisms of reinforcement. Whether a single neurotransmitter/neuroanatomical circuit will code reinforcement beyond the nucleus accumbens or whether parallel processing will continue for opiates and stimulants are questions that remain for future research.

REFERENCES

Amalric, M., Koob, G.F. (1985) Low doses of methylnaloxonium in the nucleus accumbens antagonize the hyperactivity induced by heroin in the rat. *Pharmacology Biochemistry and Behavior* 236:411–415.

Babbini, M., Davis, N.M. (1972) Time-dose relationships for locomotor activity effects of morphine after acute or repeated treatment. *Br. J. Pharmacol.* 46:213–224.

Bianchi, G., Fiocchi, R., Tavani, A., Manara, L. (1982) Quaternary narcotic antagonists relative ability to prevent antinociception and gastrointestinal transit inhibition in morphine treated rats as an index of peripheral selectivity. *Life Sci.* 30:1875–1883.

Bloom, F.E., Segal, D., Ling, N., Guillemin, R. (1976) Endorphins: Profound behavioral effects in rats suggest new etiological factors in mental illness. *Science* 194:630–632.

Bozarth, M.A., Wise, R.A. (1981a) Heroin reward is dependent on a dopaminergic substrate. *Life Sci.* 29:1881–1886.

Bozarth, M.A., Wise, R.A. (1981b) Intracranial self-administration of morphine into the ventral tegmental area in rats. *Life Sci.* 28:551–555.

Britt, M.D., Wise, R.A. (1983) Ventral tegmental site of opiate reward: antagonism by a hydrophilic opiate receptor blocker. *Brain Res.* 258:105–108.

Broekkamp, C.L.E., Phillips, A.G., Cools, A.R. (1979) Stimulant effects of enkephalin microinjection into the dopaminergic A10 area. *Nature* 278:560–562.

Bunney, W.C., Massari, V.J., Pert, A. (1984) Chronic morphine-induced hyperactivity in rats is altered by nucleus accumbens and ventral tegmental lesions. *Psychopharmacol.* 82:318–321.

Davis, W.M., Smith, S.G. (1975) Effect of haloperidol on (±)-amphetamine self-administration. *J. Pharmacol. Pharm.* 27:540–542.

Deneau, G.A., Yanagita, J., Seevers, M.H. (1969) Self-administration of psychoactive substances by the monkey. *Psychopharmacol.* 16:30–48.

DeWit, H., Wise, R.A. (1977) Blockade of cocaine reinforcement in rats with the dopamine receptor blocker pimozide, but not with the noradrenergic blockers phentolamine or phenoxybenzamine. *Canad. J. Psychol.* 31:195–203.

Ettenberg, A., Pettit, H.O., Bloom, F.E., Koob, G.F. (1982) Heroin and cocaine intravenous self-administration rats: Mediation by separate neural systems. *Psychopharmacolog.* 78:204–209.

Glickman, S.E., Schiff, B.B. (1967) A biological theory of reinforcement. *Psychol. Rev.* 74:81–108.

Goeders, N.E., Lane, J.D., Smith, J.E. (1984) Self-administration of methionine enkephalin into the nucleus accumbens. *Pharmacol. Biochem. Behav.* 20:451–455.

Goldberg, S.R., Woods, J.H., Schuster, C.R. (1971) Nalorphine-induced changes in morphine self-administration rhesus monkeys. *J. Pharmacol. Exp. Ther.* 176: 464–471.

Havemann, U., Winkler, M., Kuschinsky, K. (1983) The effects of D-ala², D-Leu⁵-enkephalin injections into the nucleus accumbens on the motility of rats. *Life Sci.* 33:627–630.

Jaffe, J.H. (1980). Drug addiction and drug abuse. In Goodman, L.S., Gilman, A., Mayer, S.E., Melmon, K.L. (eds.), *Goodman and Gilman's the Pharmacological Basis of Therapeutics.* New York: Macmillan, pp. 545–546.

Jonsson, L.E., Anggard, E., Gunne, L.M. (1971) Blockade of intravenous amphetamine euphoria in man. *Clin. Pharmacol. Ther.* 12:889–896.

Joyce, E.M., Iversen, S.D. (1979) The effect of morphine applied locally to mesencephalic dopamine cell bodies on spontaneous motor activity in the rat. *Neurosci. Lett.* 14:207–212.

Joyce, E., Koob, G.F. (1981) Amphetamine-, scopolamine, and caffeine-induced locomotor activity following 6-hydroxydopamine lesions of the mesolimbic dopamine system. *Psychopharmacol.* 73:311–313.

Joyce, E.M., Koob, G.F., Strecker, R., Iversen, S.D., Bloom, F.E. (1981) The behavioral effects of enkephalin analogues injected into the ventral tegmental area and globus pallidus. *Brain Res.* 221:359–370.

Kalivas, P.W., Widerlov, E., Stanley, D., Breese, G., Prange, Jr., A.J. (1983) Enkephalin action on the mesolimbic system: a dopamine-dependent and dopamine-independent increase in locomotor activity. *J. Pharmacol. Exp. Ther.* 227:1–9.

Kelley, A.E., Stinus, L., Iversen, S.D. (1980) Interactions between D-ala-met-enkephalin, A10 dopaminergic neurones, and spontaneous behaviour in the rat. *Behav. Brain Res.* 1:3–24.

Kelly, P.H., Seviour, P.W., Iversen, S.D. (1975) Amphetamine and apomorphine responses in the rat following 6-OHDA of the nucleus accumbens septi and corupus striatum. *Brain Res* 94: 507–522.

Koob, G.F., Bloom, F.E. (1983) Behavioral effects of opioid peptides. *Bri. Med. Bull.* 39(1):89–94.

Koob, G.F., Pettit, H.O., Ettenberg, A., Bloom, F.E. (1984) Effects of opiate antagonists and their quarternary derivatives on heroin self-administration in the rat. *J. Pharmacol. Exp. Ther.* 229:481–486.

Koob, G.F., Stinus, L., LeMoal, M. (1981) Hyperactivity and hypoactivity produced by lesions to the mesolimbic dopamine system. *Behav. Brian Res.* 3:341–359.

Koob, G.F. (1986) Separate neurochemical substrates for cocaine and heroin reinforcement. In Church, R.M., Commons, M.L. Steilar, J., and Wagner, A.R. (eds.), *Quantitative Analyses of Behavior*, Volume 7 (Hillsdale, N. J., Lawrence Erlbaum, in press).

Lyness, W.H., Friedle, N.M., Moore, K.E. (1979) Destruction of dopaminergic nerve terminals in nucleus accumbens: effect of *d*-amphetamine self-administration. *Pharmacol. Biochem. Behav.* 11:663–666.

Meyer, R.E., Mirin, S.M. (1979) *The Heroin Stimulus.* New York: Plenum, pp. 61–91.

Patrick, R.L., Snyder, T.E., Barchas, J.D. (1975) Regulation of dopamine synthesis in rat brain striatal synaptosomes. *Mol. Pharmacol.* 11:621–631.

Pert, A., Sivit, C. (1977) Neuroanatomical focus for morphine and enkephalin-induced hypermotility. *Nature* (London) 265:645–647.

Pettit, H.O., Ettenberg, A., Bloom, F.E., Koob, G.F. (1984) Destruction of the nucleus accumbens selectively attenuates cocaine but not heroin self-administration in rats. *Psychopharmacol.* 84:167–173.

Phillips, A.G., LePiane, F.G. (1980) Reinforcing effects of morphine microinjection into the ventral tegmental area. *Pharmacol. Biochem. Behav.*, 12:965–968.

Pickens, R., Harris, W.C. (1968) Self-administration of *d*-amphetamine by rats. *Psychopharmacol.* 12:158–163.

Pickens, R., Meisch, R.A., Dougherty, J.A. (1968) Chemical interactions in methamphetamine reinforcement. *Psychology Rep.* 23:1267–1270.

Pickens, R., Meisch, R.A., Thompson, J., (1978) Drug self-administration: An analysis of the reinforcing effects of drugs. In Iversen, L.L., Iversen, S.D., and Synder, S.H. (eds.), *Handbook of Psychopharmacology*, Vol. 12. New York: Plenum, pp. 1–37.

Roberts, D.C.S., Corcoran, M.E., Fibiger, H.C. (1977) On the role of ascending catecholaminergic systems in intravenous self-administration of cocaine. *Pharmacol. Biochem. Behav.* 6:615–620.

Roberts, D.C.S., Koob, G.F., Klonoff, P., Fibiger, H.C. (1980) Extinction and recovery of cocaine self-administration following 6-hydroxydopamine lesions of the nucleus accumbens. *Pharmacol. Biochem. Behav.*, 12:781–787.

Russell, J., Bass, P., Goldberg, L.J., Schuster, C.R., Merz, H. (1982) Antagonism of gut, but not central effects of morphine with quaternary narcotic antagonists. *Eur. J. Pharmacol.* 78:255–261.

Schuster, C.R., Thompson, T. (1969) Self-administration and behavioral dependence on drugs. *Annual Rev. Pharmacol.* 9:483–502.

Stinus, L., Koob, G.F., Ling, N., Bloom, F.E., LeMoal, M. (1980) Locomotor activation induced by infusion of endorphins into the ventral tegmental area: Evidence for opiate-dopamine interactions. *Proceedings of the National Academy of Sciences* (USA) 77:2323–2327.

Swerdlow, N.R., Swanson, L.W., Koob, G.F. (1984) Substantia inominata: critical link in the behavioral expression of mesolimbic dopamine stimulation. *Neuroscience Lett.* 50:19–24.

Tavani, A., Bianchi, G., Manara, L. (1979) Morphine no longer blocks gastrointestinal transit but retains antinociceptive action in diallyl-normorphine-pretreated rats. *Eur. J. Pharmacol.* 59:151–154.

Thompson, T., Pickens, R. (1970) Stimulant self-administration by animals: some comparisons with opiate self-administration. *Fed. Proc.* 29:6–11.

Vaccarino, F.J., Bloom, F.E., Koob, G.F. (1985) Blockade of nucleus accumbens opiate receptors attenuates intravenous heroin reward in the rat. *Psychopharmacol.* 86:37–42.

Vaccarino, F.J., Pettit, H.O., Bloom, F.E., Koob, G.F. (1985) Effects of intracerebroventricular administration of methylnaloxonium chloride on heroin self-administration in the rat. *Pharmacol. Biochem. Behav.* 23:495–498.

Vaccarino, F.J., Amalric, M., Swerdlow, N.R., and Koob, G.F. (1986) Blockade of amphetamine but not opiate-induced locomotion following antagonism of dopamine function in the rat. *Pharmacol. Biochem. Behav.* 24:61–65.

Valentino, R.J., Herling, S., Woods, J.H. Medizhradsky, F., Merz, H. (1981) Quarternary naltrexone: evidence for the central mediation of discriminative stimulus effects of narcotic agonists and antagonists. *J. Pharmacol. Exp. Ther.* 217:652–659.

Valentino, R.J., Katz, J.L., Medzihradsky, F., Woods, J.H. (1983) Receptor binding, antagonist and withdrawal-precipitating properties of opiate antagonists. *Life Sci.* 32:2887–2896.

Way, E.L., Adler, T.K. (1960) The pharmacologic implications of the fate of morphine and its surrogates. *Pharmacol. Rev.* 12:383–446.

Weeks, J.R., Collins, R.J. (1976) Changes in morphine self-administration in rats induced by prostagland in E and naloxone. *Prostagland.* 12:11–19.

Wikler, A. (1952) Psychodynamic study of a patient during experimental self-regulated readdiction to morphine. *Psychiatry Q.* 26:270–293.

Wise, R.A. (1982) Neuroleptics and operant behavior: the anhedonia hypothesis. *Behav. Brain Sci.* 5:39–88.

Woods, J.H., Schuster, C.R. (1968) Reinforcement properties of morphine, cocaine, and SPA as a function of unit dose. *Inter. J. Addic.* 3:231–237.

Yokel, R.A., Wise, R.A. (1976) Attenuation of intravenous amphetamine reinforcement by central dopamine blockade in rats. *Psychopharmacol.* 48:311–318.

Yokel, R.A., Pickens, R. (1973) Self-administration of optical isomers of amphetamine and methylamphetamine by rats. *J. Pharmacol. Exp. Ther.* 187:27–33.

Yokel, R.A., Wise, R.A. (1975) Increased lever pressing for amphetamine after pimozide in rats: implications for a dopamine theory of reward. *Science* 187:547–549.

Yokel, R.A., Wise, R.A. (1976) Attenuation of intravenous amphetamine reinforcement by central dopamine blockade in rats. *Psychopharmacol.* 48:311–318.

ACKNOWLEDGMENTS

This work was supported by grants 03665 from NIDA and 06420 from NIAAA. The authors thank Endo Laboratories for providing us with naloxone and the National Institute on Drug Abuse for providing the heroin and cocaine hydrochloride. We also gratefully thank Dr. Joop de Graaf of

Organon for providing us with methyl naloxonium chloride (ORG 109086). Thanks to Robert Lintz for superb technical assistance, Douglas Lee for performing the experiments reported in Figure 4.1, and Ms. Nancy Callahan for manuscript preparation. Many thanks to our colleagues Hugh Pettit, Dr. David C.S. Roberts, Dr. Aaron Ettenberg, and Dr. Floyd E. Bloom for their help and collaboration in the work reported herein.

5 | Chronic Cocaine Administration: Sensitization and Kindling Effects

ROBERT M. POST, SUSAN R.B. WEISS, AGU PERT, and THOMAS W. UHDE

STUDIES of the effects of repeated cocaine administration are required in order to interpret the clinical effects of cocaine in humans. Although patterns of administration differ markedly among individuals both in terms of route utilized and time course of repetition, cocaine use tends to be repetitive. Because of the brevity of the cocaine-induced high, repeated doses are often taken in an attempt to maintain peak mood elevation and euphoria.) At the same time, use is often intermittent because of limitations imposed by supply and cost or because of intervening periods of sleep. While there is evidence for the development of acute tolerance or tachyphylaxis with repeated administration after intervals of minutes to hours (Fischman, 1984), there is a substantial body of evidence suggesting that there may be sensitization or reverse tolerance to many effects of cocaine when administered at longer intervals (Post & Kopanda, 1976; Post et al., 1976, 1984a, Post, 1981b; Post & Ballenger, 1981; Post & Contel, 1983). In this chapter we focus on the laboratory and clinical evidence for such a sensitization effect and review possible underlying mechanisms.

Even when administered in its pure form, cocaine is a complex drug sharing major properties of at least two classes of agents. It is a potent local anaesthetic with milligram per milligram effects equal to that of local anaesthetic lidocaine (xylocaine). In contrast to the pure local anaesthetics such as lidocaine or procaine, cocaine is, in addition, a potent psychomotor stimulant sharing many behavioral and biochemical properties with the classical psychomotor stimulants amphetamine and methylphenidate (Martin et al., 1971; Fischman et al., 1976). Thus, interpretation of the effects of cocaine is complicated by its dual nature as a local anaesthetic and psychomotor stimulant. In an attempt to determine what aspects of cocaine's effects may be due solely to its local anaesthetic component, we have conducted a series of studies utilizing the local anaesthetic lidocaine given chronically to rats and the local anaesthetic procaine administered acutely (i.v.) to patients.

The psychomotor stimulant effects of cocaine are thought to be related to its ability to block reuptake of dopamine and norepinephrine (Ross & Renyi, 1966; Hertting et al., 1961; van Rossum, 1970; Scheel-Kruger et al., 1977; Kuczenski, 1983). While there is some continued controversy as to the role that potentiation of noradrenergic compared to dopaminergic systems plays in the different components of cocaine's effects on behavior, there is substantial agreement that effects on dopaminergic mechanisms are particularly important for cocaine's locomotor stimulating and reward properties (Scheel-Kruger et al., 1977; Wise, 1984). An additional focus of this chapter will be to assess the current evidence regarding dopaminergic substrates in the brain that might be responsible for different behavioral and mood-altering effects of cocaine.

The effect on dopaminergic mechanisms will be reviewed in detail, yet it should be noted that cocaine appears to influence a variety of other neurotransmitter systems that may be important to different aspects of its clinical profile. For example, Trulson and Jacobs (1979) reported that, in addition to cocaine's potent effects on blockade of serotonin reuptake, chronic administration led to long-lasting serotonin depletions and associated aspects of the serotonin syndrome. Knapp and Mandell (1976) and Ellinwood and Kilbey (1980) have also implicated serotonergic mechanisms. In addition, a specific binding site for cocaine has recently been described by several groups of investigators (Sershen et al., 1980, 1982; Reith et al., 1981, 1983, 1984; Toth-Kennedy & Hanbauer, 1983; Hanbauer p.c., 1983; Missale et al., 1984) and chronic administration of cocaine has, paradoxically, been reported to lead to upregulation of this binding site (Hanbauer p.c., 1983).

EFFECTS OF CHRONIC COCAINE ADMINISTRATION IN THE RAT

Tatum and Seevers (1929) and Downs and Eddy (1932a,b) described a syndrome of increasing excitability in response to repeated administration of the same dose of cocaine over time. In some instances, the animals began to exhibit seizures to a dose that had previously been subconvulsive. In order to replicate these early observations, we administered the same dose of cocaine (60 mg/kg, i.p.) to rats on a once-daily basis. We confirmed the earlier observations that these animals eventually developed cocaine-induced seizures to a dose that had previously been subconvulsive; the first seizure was observed after an average of 20 ±7 injections. Six of eight rats died during or following these cocaine-induced seizures (Post, 1977). Monkeys receiving repeated intermittent, subconvulsant injections of cocaine (i.p.) also showed a progressive increase in seizure susceptibility. Seizures began to be observed to a previously subconvulsant dose, and the intervals between recurrent seizures shortened (Fig.5.1). These data contrast with those of Matsuzaki et al., (1976), also in the rhesus primate, where repeated administration of convulsant doses of cocaine (i.v.) was not associated with a change in the minimum convulsant dose.

To assess whether seizure sensitization to subconvulsant doses was related to cocaine's local anaesthetic compared to psychomotor stimulant properties, we administered equal doses of the nonpsychomotor stimulant lidocaine on a once-daily basis in the rat. Again, across many series of studies (Post et al., 1975, 1979, 1984; Post, 1981a), we observed a similar phenomenon in which initially nonconvulsant doses eventually resulted in seizures of increasing frequency, duration, and complexity (Figs. 5.2 and 5.3). However, in contrast to rats given repeated cocaine administration, these animals appeared to tolerate the seizures quite well and survived multiple episodes of seizures that often lasted, in intermittent episodes, for periods of 20 to 45 minutes and, in rare instances, several hours. We noticed that the time course of deveolopment of these seizures (Fig. 5.3) and the behavioral manifestations were strikingly similar to that observed following electrical kindling of the amygdala (Goddard et al., 1969).

In electrical kindling of the amygdala, originally described by Goddard and associates (1969), subjects received repeated once-daily

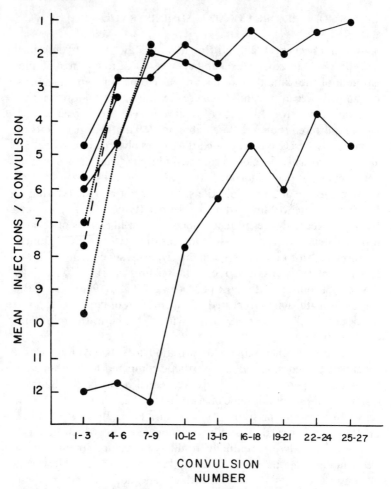

FIGURE 5.1. Increase in seizure susceptibility in monkeys following repeated administration of initially subconvulsant doses of cocaine (see Post et al., 1976). Monkeys received daily cocaine injections that eventually resulted in motor seizures with a progressive decrease in the interval between successive seizures. Each line on the figure represents a single monkey.

stimulation of the amygdala for as short a time as one second. Initially, little effect on electrical activity or behavior was seen, but eventually afterdischarges of increasing duration, spread, and complexity were produced and major motor seizures involving clonic

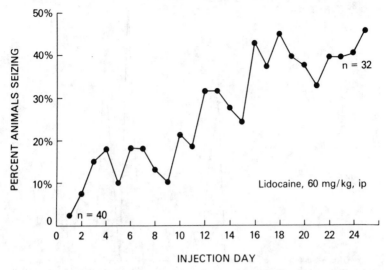

FIGURE 5.2. Progressive increase in seizure susceptibility in rats following repeated administration of an initially subconvulsive dose of lidocaine (60 mg/kg). Eight of the original 40 rats died by the 25th day of injections.

movements of the head, trunk, and forepaws with rearing and falling were also observed (Table 5.1). Since it has been well established that local anaesthetics alter amygdala electrical activity and produce a series of spike after-discharges and frank seizures, we postulated that the effects of cocaine and the pure local anaesthetics might involve a "pharmacological" kindling of the amygdala (Post et al., 1975; Post & Kopanda, 1976). Ellinwood and associates (1977) also independently suggested that a kindling-like mechanism could account for some aspects of the behavioral and convulsive sensitization to repeated cocaine administration.

One of the potential criticisms of our "pharmacological" kindling hypothesis was the possibility that repeated drug administration was leading to accumulation of local anaesthetics or their metabolites in the brain, rather than producing a true sensitization effect. A variety of indirect data suggest that this was unlikely. Cocaine has a short half-life, yet the sensitization effects are long-lasting. Preliminary data from chronic administration of cocaine in the rhesus monkey suggested that cerebrospinal fluid levels of cocaine were not different following acute and chronic administration (Post, 1977), and the cocaine half-life may decrease (Matsuzaki et al., 1976), although

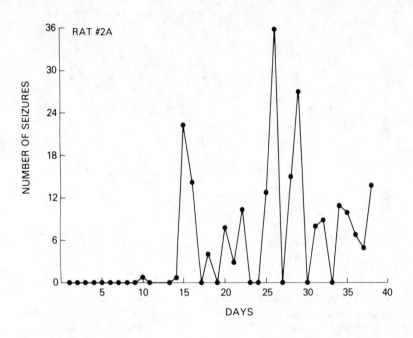

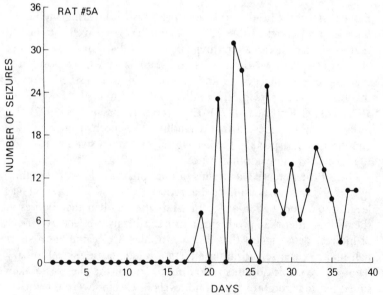

FIGURE 5.3. The pattern of onset of lidocaine-induced seizures in four individual rats is illustrated. Animals showed no seizures for one to two

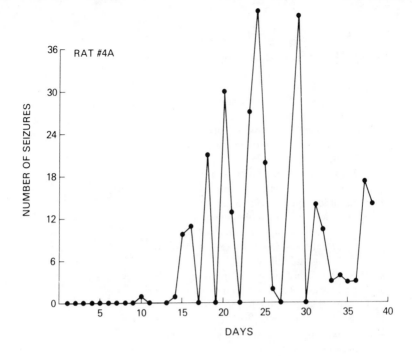

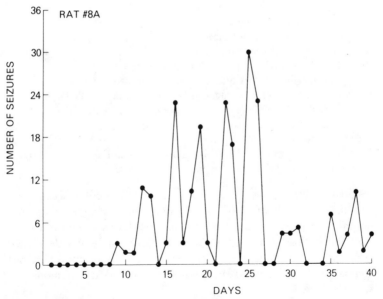

weeks and then developed intermittent seizures of varying intensity and duration.

Table 5.1 Electrical Kindling: Major Characteristics*

---

1. Repeated stimulations
   a. Initially subseizure threshold
   b. Intermittent
2. Local after-discharges and seizure activity
   a. Increases in amplitude, frequency
   b. Increase in duration
   c. Increase in complexity of wave form
   d. Increase in anatomical spread
3. Replicable sequence of seizure stages
   Behavioral arrest, blinking and masticatory
   movements, head nodding, opsithotonis,
   contralateral then bilateral forelimb clonus,
   rearing and falling
4. Discharges kindle in quantum jumps
5. Limbic system kindles more readily than cortex
6. In kindled animals the history of convulsion
   development is recapitulated as seizure builds
7. Transfer effects to secondary sites; kindling facilitated
   in other sites even after primary site destroyed
8. Interference: A secondary kindled site interferes with
   primary site rekindling
9. No toxic or neuropathological changes evident;
   kindling is a transsynaptic process
10. Relatively permanent change in connectivity; a kindled
    animal will still seize after a 1-year seizure-free interval
11. Seizure may develop spontaneously in chronically kindled animals
12. Interictal spikes and spontaneous epileptiform potentials develop

---

*See Goddard et al. (1969) regarding 1,4–10; Wada and Sato (1974)
regarding 2–4,6; Wada et al. (1974) regarding 10–12; Racine (1978); and
Pinel and Rovner (1978a,b).

residual levels in the brain have been described a week after
administration (Misra, 1976). In addition, chronic administration of
lidocaine in the rat did not appear to increase levels of lidocaine or its
metabolite (Post et al., 1984). In fact, the animals that developed
lidocaine-induced seizures had lower levels of lidocaine in plasma
compared to similarly treated animals that did not demonstrate
seizures (Fig. 5.4).

In a further attempt to more directly rule out a pharmacokinetic
alteration, we treated animals with chronic lidocaine or saline and

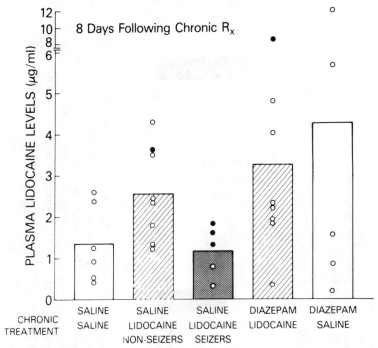

FIGURE 5.4. Recurrent lidocaine seizures are not due to increased plasma lidocaine levels. Each bar on the figure represents the group mean plasma lidocaine level following an acute lidocaine injection 45 days after chronic pretreatment. The circles illustrate the individual levels for each rat and filled circles indicate the occurrence of a motor seizure. The animals were exposed to pretreatment with diazepam (1 mg/kg) or saline followed by a lidocaine (65 mg/kg) or saline injection, in order to assess the development of lidocaine-induced seizures (see text and Fig. 5.5 for details). The animals that developed seizures during chronic lidocaine administration had similar levels to saline pretreated animals or lower levels of lidocaine in plasma compared to lidocaine-treated animals that did not develop seizures. These data suggest that the development of lidocaine seizures was not the result of increased lidocaine levels following repeated injections.

concomitantly pretreated half of the animals in each group with diazepam. Diazepam inhibits the expression of lidocaine seizures and we postulated that if chronic administration were in fact inducing a pharmacological kindling effect, it would require repeated activation of appropriate brain substrates. However, if only repeated lidocaine

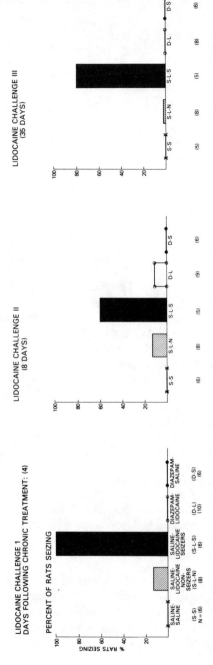

FIGURE 5.5 Seizures are necessary for lidocaine kindling; effect is blocked by diazepam co-treatment. This figure illustrates the effect of an acute lidocaine challenge 4, 8, and 35 days following or four weeks (5 times/week) with once-daily injections of lidocaine (65 mg/kg, i.p.) or saline with or without diazepam (1 mg/kg). None of the rats that received diazepam co-treatment developed lidocaine seizures, while 6 of 14 rats that received saline and lidocaine developed seizures during the chronic treatment phase of the experiment. The upper portion of the figure shows the percentage of rats in each group that seized and the lower portion of the figure shows the seizure duration. Following acute administration of lidocaine alone, seizures were seen

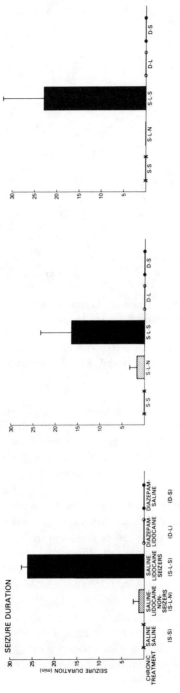

only in the lidocaine pretreated animals that did not receive diazepam co-treatment. This effect persisted when rats were rechallenged with lidocaine alone 8 and 35 days later (Pitem, Contel, Post, unpublished data). These data indicate that lidocaine-induced seizure sensitization required repeated physiological activation by lidocaine and does not occur with lidocaine plus diazepam (i.e., when the proconvulsant effects are blocked). These findings and the persistent seizure sensitization 35 days after chronic lidocaine administration was terminated support the interpretation that lidocaine is producing a bona-fide pharmacological kindling effect.

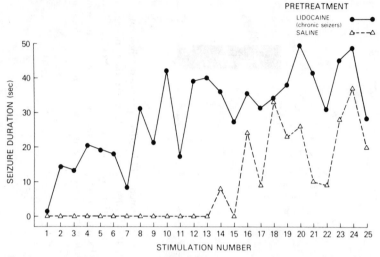

FIGURE 5.6. Lidocaine seizures facilitate the rate of amygdala kindling. The number of electrical stimulations are plotted on the abscissa and the group mean seizure duration on the ordinate. Lidocaine-kindled animals required only 5.2 ± 1.2 stimulations before exhibiting stage 4 seizures; whereas the saline-pretreated group required 18.3 ± 2.4 stimulations ($t = 5.2$, d.f. $= 7$, $p < .01$).

administration were required to somehow affect pharmacokinetic parameters or brain levels, concomitant treatment with diazepam to block the electrical excitability effects of lidocaine would still be sufficient to produce seizure sensation. When animals were rechallenged with lidocaine 8 and 35 days following termination of chronic lidocaine (and diazepam) injections, we observed (Fig. 5.5) that seizure sensitization was only present in animals that received chronic lidocaine injections without diazepam pretreatment, thus confirming that repeated activation of appropriate brain substrates was necessary for the lidocaine-induced kindling effect. These data also indicate the long-lasting nature of the altered response based on prior "effective" exposure; the increased responsivity lasted at least 35 days.

Moreover, in another study, animals experiencing repeated lidocaine-induced seizures subsequently showed faster development of electrically kindled seizures from the amygdala (Fig. 5.6), suggesting some overlapping substrates for these two types of seizures. Studies of regional glucose utilization employing deoxyglucose also

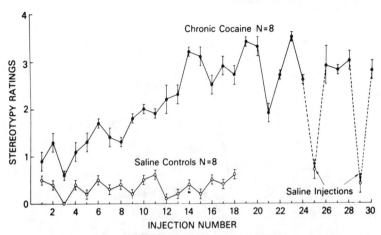

FIGURE 5.7. Increasing effect of repetitive cocaine injections on stereotypic behavior. Rats treated with cocaine (10 mg/kg, i.p.) develop progressively more intense and constricted behavioral stereotypic patterns including corner-to-corner motor sequences, vertical rearing and nose poking, and head bobbing.

indicate that the amygdala and the hippocampus and associated limbic system structures show increased metabolic activity during lidocaine-induced seizures, which are also followed by long-lasting behavioral consequences, that is, irritability and aggression (Post et al., 1984).

COCAINE-INDUCED BEHAVIORAL SENSITIZATION

A wealth of data, reviewed in detail elsewhere (Post, 1981b; Post et al., 1984b), indicates that repeated low doses of cocaine and related psychomotor stimulants in many different animal species can produce increasing behavioral effects (weeks to months as illustrated in Fig. 5.8) to the same dose (Fig. 5.7). This sensitization effect is long-lasting and related to dose (Shuster et al., 1977), gender (Post & Contel, 1983; see Figs. 5.9a, 5.9b), and genetic strain (Shuster et al., 1977). Sensitization is subject to environmental context effects and appears to involve conditioning (Post et al., 1981a; Hinson & Poulos, 1981). Eichler et al. (1980) and Rebec and Segal (1980) have emphasized that different componments of amphetamine-induced behaviors would show sensitization or tolerance; this may also be the case for cocaine. Eichler et al. found that stereotypic licking to

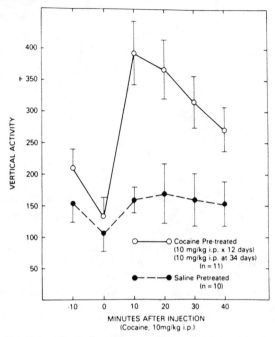

FIGURE 5.8. Long-lasting persistence of behavioral sensitization to cocaine 87 days following the termination of chronic cocaine administration. Time (pre- and post-injection) is plotted on the abscissa and vertical activity is plotted on the ordinate. Rats were pretreated for 12 days with either cocaine (10 mg/kg) or saline injections (i.p.). When challenged with an acute cocaine injection 87 days following the termination of chronic cocaine, the cocaine-pretreated animals continued to exhibit much greater activity than saline-pretreated controls.

amphetamine (8 and 12 mg/kg) showed tolerance over a two-week period, but re-emereged after day 24, at which time low doses (2 to 4 mg/kg, which had failed to elicit this behavior acutely) also produced licking. Stereotyped sniffing only showed sensitization. Rebec and Segal (1980) noted sensitization to head and limb movements, but not to oral stereotypies induced by amphetamine. Side-to-side head nodding is a prominent effect of chronic cocaine; nodding, increasingly constricted stereotypies, and immobilization appear to be late effects following chronic administration.

A variety of other endpoints, in addition to locomotor hyperactivity and stereotypy, have been shown to be sensitive to cocaine or related stimulant-induced sensitization. These include hyperthermia (Tatum & Seevers, 1929; Gutierrez-Noriga & Zapata-Ortiz, 1944), catalepsy or behavioral inhibition (Gutierrez-Noriega, 1950; Post et al., 1977) and dyskinesias (Post et al., 1977).

In addition, cocaine-induced behavioral sensitization, like several other models of learning and memory, including the development of tolerance, appears to be modulated by vasopressin (Post et al., 1982). Brattleboro homozygote rats, which are deficient in vasopressin, show a deficient onset and maintenance of cocaine-induced behavioral sensitization compared with Brattleboro heterozygotes, which have almost normal vasopressin and do not show diabetes insipidus (Figs. 5.10a, 5.10b). Replacement of homozygotes with vasopressin normalizes the defect in onset and maintenance of cocaine-induced behavioral sensitization (Post & Contel, unpublished data) (Fig. 5.10b).

The environmental context or conditioning component to cocaine-induced behavioral sensitization is noteworthy in its own right, but is also of potential clinical relevance. Based on the initial observations that animals injected with cocaine in their home cage showed less robust behavioral sensitization than animals repeatedly injected in the same environment (i.e., test cages) (Fig. 5.11), we conducted a more systematic study of this phenomenon. (Post et al., 1981a). Two groups of animals were studied. The first group received an injection of cocaine in the plexiglas test cage, were monitored for the next 40 minutes, and then received an injection of saline upon leaving the test cage. The second group received identical handling and injections, differing only in the order of saline and cocaine. The second group thus received saline in the test cage and experienced cocaine-induced hyperactivity elsewhere (i.e., in its wire home cage). As illustrated in Figure 5.12, animals treated with cocaine in the context of the test cage showed increases in degree of cocaine-induced hyperactivity as well as in ratings of stereotypy (not illustrated). On day 11, both groups of animals were injected with cocaine in the test cage. As is evident on this day and more prominently on days 13 and 14, animals repeatedly injected with cocaine in the context of the test cage were markedly more active than animals receiving identical doses of cocaine in a different environment. Following injections with saline on day 12, animals pretreated with cocaine in the test cage were also significantly more active than animals that had received cocaine in their home cages.

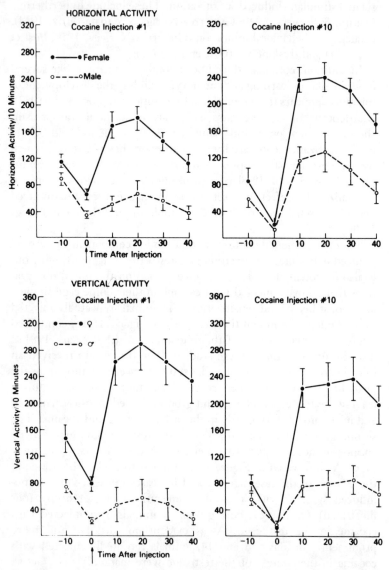

FIGURE 5.9a. Sex differences in the development of cocaine sensitization. The ordinate on each graph shows horizontal or vertical activity recorded for 20 minutes prior to and 40 minutes following cocaine injections (10 mg/kg, i.p.). Activity on days 1, 10, 16, and 20 (one week following chronic

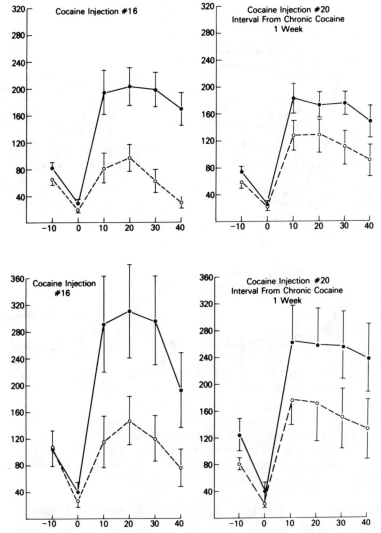

cocaine termination) is shown. The female rats (solid lines and filled circles) showed greater hyperactivity in response to the cocaine on day 1 than did male rats (broken lines and unfilled circles) and thus did not manifest a sensitization response because of "ceiling effects."

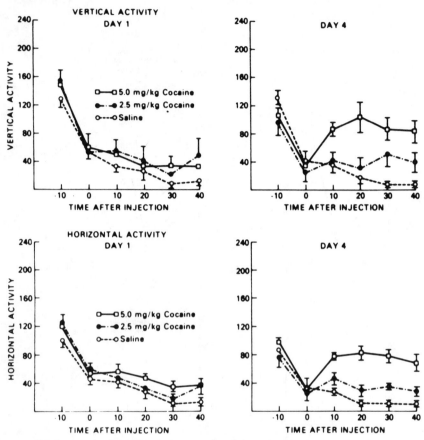

FIGURE 5.9b. The development of cocaine sensitization in female rats following repeated i.p. injections of low doses of cocaine (2.5 and 5.0 mg/kg). Horizontal and vertical activity are plotted on the ordinate of each graph and time (pre- and post-injection) is plotted on the abscissa. Since the female rats were so reactive to the dose of cocaine used to produce sensitization in male rats (10 mg/kg) and failed to show sensitization to this

However, the saline injection was not associated with marked increases in activity.

These data are supportive of the earlier observations of Ellinwood and Kilbey (1975) indicating that cats show conditional aspects of stereotypic behavior to amphetamine depending on handling and environmental context. Hinson and Poulos (1981) also documented

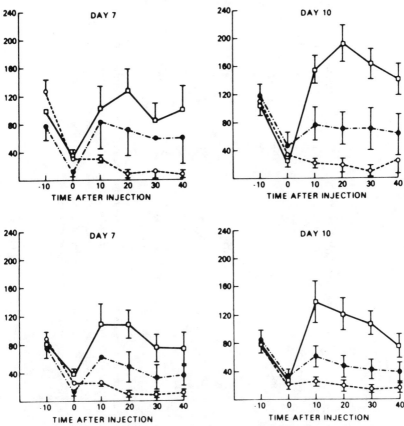

dose (see Fig. 5.9a), lower doses of cocaine were tried in an attempt to demonstrate that female rats could become sensitized to the hyperactivity produced by cocaine. The increase in locomotor activity from day 1 to day 10 following the 5.0 mg/kg dose of cocaine illustrates that female rats do show behavioral sensitization to cocaine when the appropriate dose is chosen.

the conditioned component of cocaine sensitization and have extended these findings, by showing that repeated administration of saline could desensitize or decondition this response. Schiff and Bridger (1978) demonstrated stimulant-induced conditioned behavior and amphetamine-conditioned homovanillic acid (HVA) alterations in the nucleus accumbens using conditioned stimuli, such as lights and tones.

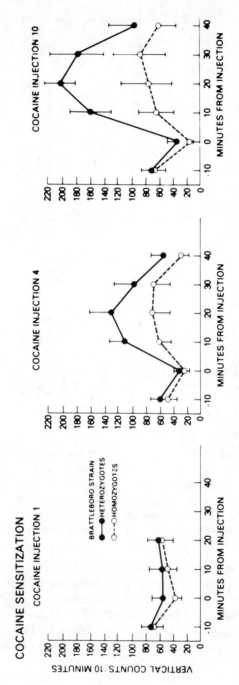

FIGURE 5.10a Impaired development of cocaine sensitization in Brattleboro rats following repeated i.p. injections of cocaine (10 mg/kg). Vertical activity counts are plotted on the ordinate of each graph and time (pre- and post-interjection) is plotted on the abscissa. Heterozygote Brattleboro rats, which are not markedly vasopression-deficient, show normal development or persistence of cocaine sensitization. In contrast, the vasopression-deficient homozygotes failed to demonstrate increased reactivity to cocaine following 10 days of administration or on subsequent challenges.

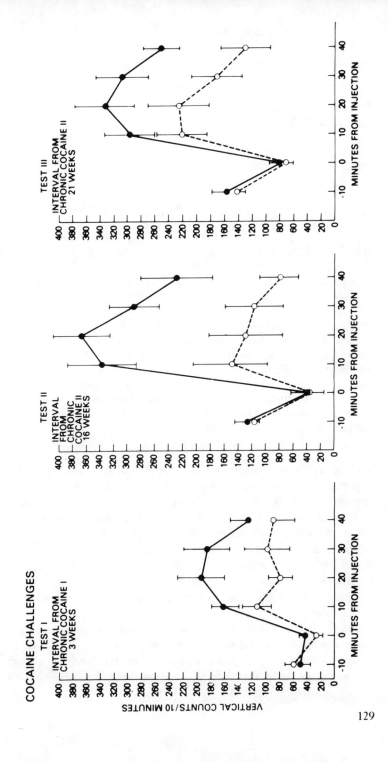

129

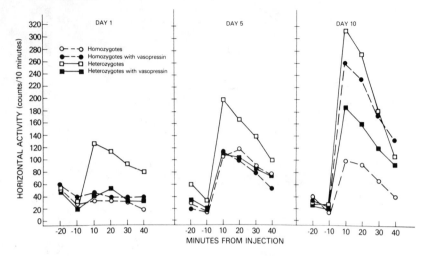

FIGURE 5.10b. Effect of vasopressin replacement on cocaine sensitization in homozygote Brattleboro rates. As Figure 5.10a illustrates, impaired cocaine sensitization was observed in vasopressin-deficient Brattleboro rats. Administration of pitressin (.1 mg/100g, i.p., 2 hours prior to cocaine) resulted in the development of normal cocaine sensitization by the homozygote Brattleboro rats. The vaspressin treatment itself did not enhance cocaine-induced locomotor activity, as can be seen in heterozygotes that received vasopressin co-treatment.

Using a different paradigm, Collins et al. (1979) demonstrated the importance of environmental context and cueing in subsequent responsivity to cocaine. They showed that cocaine administration could lead to either increased or decreased responding, dependent on prior stimulus associations. Woolverton et al. (1978) reported tolerance to the effects of cocaine repeatedly administered prior to the availability of a sweetened milk solution; but when chronic cocaine was administered after milk (postsession), rats were more sensitive to the suppressive effects of acute presession cocaine on milk intake.

These data in animals offer many possible explanations for differences in behavioral responsivity to a given dose of cocaine in humans. Prior drug experience and its context and behavioral contingencies could alter affective and behavioral responsivity, in

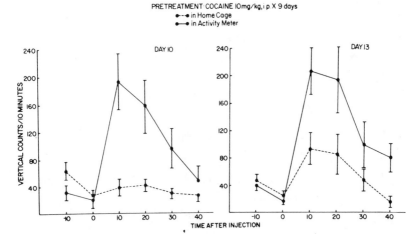

FIGURE 5.11. Effect of home cage vs. activity meter cage in cocaine-treated rats. Rats treated repeatedly with cocaine (10 mg/kg i.p. once daily) in the activity meter cage show significantly greater activity than those treated with the same dose in their home cage and challenged with cocaine in the activity meter cage on days 10 and 13. Note the increased activity in the home-cage-treated animals following their second cocaine injection in the meter (day 13 compared to day 10). These findings of an environment context component to behavior are not related to the degree of prior exposure to apparatus in the absence of drug effect, but appear to depend on the occurrence of cocaine-induced activity in a given context (Post et al., 1981a). Animals receiving repeated injections of saline in the activity meter and cocaine injections upon leaving it also show less cocaine-induced activity than animals receiving identical experience and treatment, but injections in the reverse order (i.e., cocaine in the activity meter, saline upon leaving).

addition to the more usually considered variables of dose, route, and speed of administration, interval between injections, sex, temperature, initial mood or behavioral state, and degree of activation, as well as individual differences in drug susceptibility and metabolism. The data on the context-dependency of cocaine-induced sensitization (Figs. 5.11, 5.12, 5.13) also eliminate the possibility that pharmacokinetic alterations account for the sensitization, as both groups of animals had identical cocaine doses.

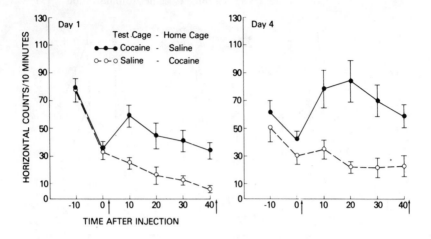

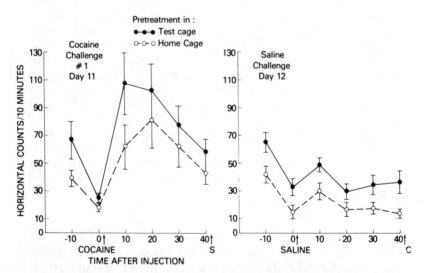

FIGURE 5.12. *Top:* Cocaine pretreatment in different environmental contexts; cocaine sensitization. *Bottom:* Effect of environmental context on cocaine sensitization. Increasing motor response to once-daily cocaine (10 mg/kg, i.p.) is observed only in test cage-treated animals (days 1–10). Moreover, test-cage-treated animals showed greater motor activity follow-

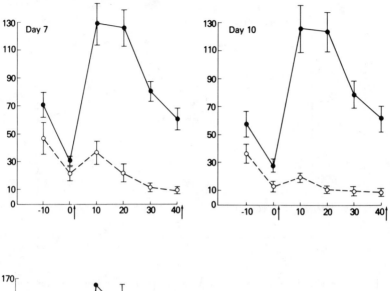

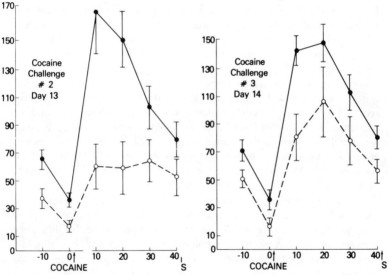

ing cocaine challenge #2 ($p<0.01$) and #3 ($p<0.05$) than animals that received the same number of previous cocaine doses, but in their home cage. Test-cage-treated animals were also more active before and after saline challenge (day 12) than those treated in their home cage ($p<0.001$). These data support a role for conditioning variables in cocaine-induced behavioral sensitization.

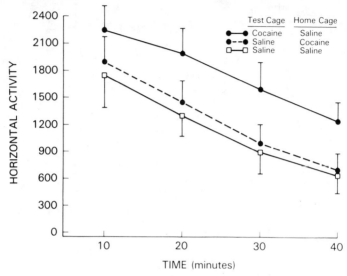

FIGURE 5.13a. Increased response to an amphetamine injection into the nucleus accumbens following chronic cocaine in the same environment. Three groups of rats received daily i.p. injections of cocaine (10 mg/kg) or saline for 10 days. One injection was given just prior to being placed in the test chamber in which activity was being measured, and the second injection occurred when the rats were returned to the home cage. One group received cocaine in the test environment and saline in the home cage; a second group received saline in the test environment and cocaine in the home cage; and the third group received two saline injections. Following this chronic regimen an acute challenge with amphetamine (10 μg) injected directly into the nucleus accumbens bilaterally revealed a significant difference ($F = 3.19$, $p < .09$; one-tailed ANOVA with repeated measures) in the locomotor activity exhibited by the rats that previously received cocaine in the test chamber and those that had never received cocaine. These differences could, however, be accounted for by the differences in baselines of the two groups (see Fig. 5.13b) as opposed to a difference in their sensitivity to amphetamine. No difference between the rats that received cocaine in the home cage and those that had never received cocaine was seen, further emphasizing the strength of the conditioning or context dependency component of this behavior.

POTENTIAL MECHANISMS FOR COCAINE-INDUCED BEHAVIORAL SENSITIZATION

A list of potential candidates for important mechanisms underlying behavioral sensitization is presented in Table 5.2 There is strong

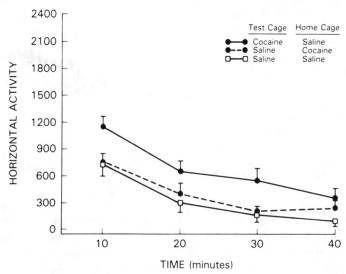

FIGURE 5.13b. Increased response to a saline injection into the nucleus accumbens following chronic cocaine in the same environment. Rats received daily i.p. injections of cocaine (10 mg/kg) in the test or home cage (as described in Fig. 5.14). Following this chronic regimen and 5 days after the amphetamine challenge, an acute challenge with saline injected directly into the nucleus accumbens revealed a significant ($F = 7.79, p < .02$; ANOVA with repeated measures) increase in the locomotor activity exhibited by the rats that previously received cocaine in the test chamber and those that had never received cocaine, suggesting a strong environmental context or conditioning effect of the cocaine pretreatment in the test environment.

evidence that the acute effects of cocaine on locomotor activity depend on dopaminergic activity in the nucleus accumbens (Kelly & Iversen, 1976). Thus, it remains a possibility that alterations in dopaminergic activity in this area of brain could underlie stimulant-induced behavioral sensitization (Table 5.3). Nucleus accumbens lesions also block cocaine self-administration (Roberts et al., 1980; Pettit et al., 1984). The mesocortical dopamine systems may also be involved in some aspects of cocaine-reinforced behavior as this area, but not the nucleus accumbens, supports intracranial self-administration (Goeders & Smith, 1983) and 6-hydroxydopamine lesions of the medial prefrontal cortex disrupt this self-administration (Goeders & Smith, 1984) as well as cocaine-reinforced place prefer-

Table 5.2 Possible Mechanisms for Behavioral Sensitization to Cocaine

---

Pharmacodynamics
Catecholamine depletion supersensitivity
Serotonin, GABA imbalances
Increase post-synaptic DA receptors
Presynaptic DA receptor desensitization
  (Increased presynaptic release)
Endocrine and peptide modulation
Increased [^{3}H]-cocaine binding
  (regionally selective)
Local anaesthetic and kindling-like effects

---

ence (Isaac et al., 1984). Medial prefrontal cortex lesions do not disrupt intravenous cocaine self-administration (Szostak et al., 1984), further supporting a role for other brain structures, such as the nucleus accumbens, in this type of behavior.

Moreover, while many studies of ^{3}H-spiroperidol binding following chronic stimulant administration (with amphetamine) tend to show no change or decreases in straitum (Table 5.4), several reports have indicated that this measure of dopamine receptor binding may increase in nucleus accumbens (Howlett & Nahorski, 1978; Robert, 1979; Akiyama et al., 1982a,b; Wirz-Justice, 1983). However, Hitzemann et al. (1980) and Ridley et al. (1982) reported decreased binding in the nucleus accumbens after amphetamine. Thus, it remains a possibility to be confirmed with direct testing whether alterations in dopamine receptor binding might occur in nucleus accumbens following chronic cocaine administration.

In an attempt to directly assess whether chronic cocaine produced alterations in dopamine receptor sensitivity in either nucleus accumbens or caudate nucleus, we treated groups of animals with cocaine (10 mg/kg) or saline once daily for 10 days and then challenged them with amphetamine (10 μg) and saline (1 μl) injected into nucleus accumbens bilaterally. In order to further evaluate the effect of conditioning, the cocaine treated animals received the drug either in the context of their test cage or in their home cage. The results of this study indicate that animals repeatedly treated with cocaine in the test cage have greater locomotor activity in response to both saline or amphetamine injected into the nucleus accumbens than do the other two groups (i.e., chronic saline-injected animals or animals treated

Table 5.3 Regional Dopaminergic Substrates of cocaine

Striatum	N. Accumbens	Mesocortical
	6-OHDA lesions: ↓ *Motor activity* (Kelly & Iversen, 1975)	*Intracranial self-administration into medial prefrontal ctx,* not N. Acc., not VTA (Goeders & Smith, 1983)
	6-OHDA lesions: ↓ *Self-administration* (Roberts et al., 1980)	6-OHDA lesions: ↓ *intracranial self-administration to medial prefrontal ctx* (Goeders & Smith, 1984)
	↓ *Self-administration of cocaine, not heroin* (Petti et al., 1984)	Suction lesions: ↓ *cocaine-reinforced conditioned place preference* (Isacc et al., 1984)
		6-OHDA lesions: *Not disrupt cocaine self administration (i.v.)* (Szostak et al., 1984)
Cocaine dose-related Potent block of DA uptake (ut)		*Weak block of DA uptake* (Hadfield & Nugent, 1983)
Cocaine (20 mg/kg,i.p.) ×1 day ↓ *DA uptake 35%*	↑ *DA uptake 40%*	
Cocaine (20 mg/kg,i.p.) ×21 days *Tolerance (to* ↓ *DA ut)* $IC_{50} = 10$ uM	*No tolerance (to* ↓ *DA ut)* $IC_{50} = 100$ uM	
Na+ dependent *[3H]-cocaine binding*	*Not detectable* *[3H]-cocaine binding* (Missale et al., 1984)	
[3H]-cocaine binding stimulated by 25-50 mM Na+ *Related to DA uptake*	*[3H]-cocaine binding (Non-Na+ sensitive) Related to serotonin uptake* (Reith et al., 1984)	

Table 5.4a Receptor Binding Effects of Stimulants and Related Compounds
Evidence for Receptor Increases

Species, Tissue	Treatment	Duration	Receptor Ligand binding	Investigators
Calf caudate homogenate	Dopamine Norepinephrine	1 hr. incubation	↑ [^{3}H] apomorphine No change [^{3}H]-WB-4101 No change ,[^{3}H] naloxone	McManus et al., 1978
Rat limbic, rat striatum	Dopamine or Bromocriptine	½ hr. incubation	↑ [^{3}H] apomorphine	Robertson, 1980
Rat striatum	L-DOPA	Chronic	↑[^{3}H] dopamine	Klawans et al., 1977a,b
Rat striatum	L-DOPA	11 days	↑[^{3}H] spiroperidol	Wilner et al., 1980
Rat striatum	L-DOPA	6 months	↑[^{3}H] spiroperidol ↑[^{3}H] 5-HT ↑[^{3}H] ADTN	Pycock et al., 1982
Guinea pig striatum	L-DOPA	3 weeks	↑[^{3}H] dopamine	Hitri & Klawans, 1978
Rat striatum	Amphetamine	5 weeks	↑[^{3}H] dopamine	Borison et al., 1979
Rat striatum	Amphetamine	single injection	↑[^{3}H] pimozide	Baudry et al., 1977
Rat striatum	Amphetamine	6 weeks	↑[^{3}H] aloprenolol	Banerjee et al., 1978
Guinea pig striatum	Amphetamine	4 weeks	↑[^{3}H] dopamine ↑ affinity	Klawans et al., 1979
Rat limbic	Amphetamine	4, 20 days	↑[^{3}H] spiperone	Howlett & Nahorski, 1978

Tissue	Drug	Duration	Effect	Reference
Rat limbic, rat striatum	Amphetamine	22 days	↑ $[^3\text{H}]$ spiroperidol (in both areas)	Robertson, 1979
Rat limbic	Amphetamine	14 days, single injection	↑ $[^3\text{H}]$ spiperone	Akiyama et al., 1982b
Rat limbic	Amphetamine	14 days	↑ $[^3\text{H}]$ spiperone (high affinity site only)	Akiyama et al., 1982a
Rat limbic	Amphetamine	weeks	↑ $[^3\text{H}]$ spiroperidol	Wirz-Justice, 1983
Guinea pig striatum	Amphetamine	3 weeks	↑ $[^3\text{H}]$ dopamine	Hitri & Klawans, 1978
Rat striatum	Cocaine	5 weeks	↑ $[^3\text{H}]$ dopamine	Borison et al., 1979
Rat striatum	Cocaine	6 weeks	↑ $[^3\text{H}]$ aloprenolol	Chanda et al., 1979
Rat striatum	Cocaine	3 weeks	↑ $[^3\text{H}]$ aloprenolol, ↑ $[^3\text{H}]$-WB-4101	Part et al., 1979
Rat striatum	Cocaine	single injection	↑ $[^3\text{H}]$ spiroperidol, ↑ $[^3\text{H}]$ N-propylnorapomorphine	Memo et al., 1981
Rat striatum	Cocaine	single injection	↑ $[^3\text{H}]$ spiroperidol	Hanbauer et al., 1981
Rat striatum	Cocaine	1 and 2 weeks	↑ $[^3\text{H}]$ spiroperidol	Taylor et al, 1979
Rat striatum	Cocaine	6 weeks, single injection	↑ $[^3\text{H}]$ dihydroalprenolol	Banerjee et al, 1979
Rat limbic, rat striatum	PEA	22 days	↑ $[^3\text{H}]$ spiroperidol (in both areas)	Robertson, 1979

Table 5.4b Receptor Binding Effects of Stimulants and Related Compounds
Lack of Evidence for Receptor Increases

Species, Tissue	Treatment	Duration	Receptor Ligand binding	Investigators
Rat striatum	L-Dopa	10 days	Reversal of ↑ [³H] dopamine with haloperidol	Friedhoff et al., 1977
Mouse limbic, mouse striatum	L-Dopa	9 months	No change [³H] spiroperidol	Sahakian et al., 1980
Rat striatum	L-Dopa and benserazide	12 days	No change [³H] spiperone [³H] leu-enkephalin	Jackson et al., 1983
Rat striatum	Bromocriptine	2-7 days	↓ [³H] spiperone (25-50%)	Quik & Iverson, 1978
Rat striatum	Bromocriptine	7 days	No change [³H] spiperone	Globus et al., 1982
Rat striatum	Amphetamine	3 weeks	No change [³H] haloperidol	Burt et al., 1977
Rat striatum	Amphetamine or apomorphine	14 days 14 days	↓ [³H] apomorphine No change [³H] haloperidol	Muller Seeman, 1979
Rat striatum	Amphetamine	20 days (not 4)	↓ [³H] spiroperidol	Howlett & Nahorski, 1979
Rat striatum	Amphetamine	25 days	No change [³H] spiperone	Jackson et al., 1981

140

Region/Species	Drug	Duration	Effect	Reference
Rat striatum frontal cortex	Amphetamine	5 days	↓ [³H] spiroperidol ↓ [³H]LSD	Nielson et al., 1980
Rat striatum	Amphetamine	7 days	No change [³H] haloperidol	Algieri et al., 1980
Rat limbic rat striatum	Amphetamine	4 days	↑ [³H] spiroperidol	Hitzemann et al., 1980
Rat striatum	Amphetamine	4, 20 days	↓ [³H] spiperone	Howlett & Nahorski, 1978
Rat striatum	Amphetamine	14 days single injection	↓ [³H] spiperone	Akiyama et al., 1982
Rat striatum	Amphetamine	14 days	↓ [³H] spiperone (high affinity site only)	Akiyama et al., 1982
Rat striatum	Amphetamine	weeks	No change [³H] spiroperidol	Wirz-Justice, 1983
Guinea pig striatum	Amphetamine	3 weeks	↓ [³H] dopamine	Hitri & Klawans, 1978
Mouse striatum	Amphetamine N-n-propylnorapomorphine Apomorphine	14 days	↓ [³H] spiroperidol ↓ [³H] spiroperidol No change	Riffee et al., 1982
Monkey accumbens, monkey striatum	Amphetamine	35 days	↓ [³H] spiperone (not significant; 50% in accumbens)	Ridley et al, 1982
Monkey caudate	Amphetamine	35 days	No change [³H] spiperone	Owen et al, 1980

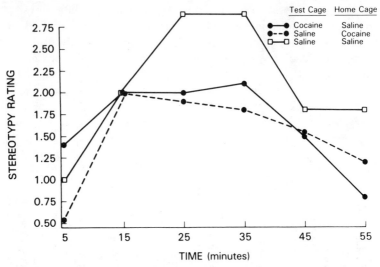

FIGURE 5.14. Lack of effect of prior cocaine treatment on amphetamine-induced stereotypy following caudate injection. Three groups of rats received 2 daily i.p. injections of cocaine or saline for a total of 17 days. Stereotypy ratings were made using a modified version of the Creese and Iverson scale (1974) at 10-minute intervals beginning 5 minutes after the injection and lasting for 55 minutes post-injection. The group mean ratings are plotted on the ordinate and time is plotted on the abscissa. The dose of cocaine used for the first 10 days was 10 mg/kg and for the last 7 days was 20 mg/kg. Saline was always administered in a volume of 1 ml/kg (which was equivalent to the volume of cocaine). One injection was given to the rats just prior to being placed in the test cage in which stereotypy was rated and a second injection occurred when the rats were returned to the home cage. One group received cocaine in the test environment and saline in the home cage; a second group received saline in the test environment and cocaine in the home cage; and the third group received two saline injections. Following this chronic regimen, an acute challenge with amphetamine injected directly into the caudate revealed no significant differences among the three groups, although the cocaine pretreated groups (regardless of location or injection) showed slightly less stereotypic behavior.

with identical doses of cocaine but in the different environmental context of their home cage) (Fig. 5.13a,b). These data indicate that there is a robust environmental context effect revealed under either saline or amphetamine in the animals treated with cocaine in the same test environment challenge conditions. However, differences in activity following saline would appear to account for differences in response to amphetamine injected into the nucleus accumbens.

Another series of rats prepared with bilateral caudate cannulae were injected in the caudate with amphetamine and cocaine following 17 days of i.p. cocaine or saline pretreatment. Cocaine pretreated animals had nonsignificantly decreased levels of stereotypy compared to saline controls following amphetamine (Fig. 5.14) and equivalent levels of stereotypy following cocaine (data not shown). Interestingly, the cocaine injected into the caudate produced identical patterns of stereotypic behavior to systemically injected cocaine in the cocaine-pretreated animals, further suggesting a role of the caudate in cocaine-induced stereotypy. Even so, no enhancement of the stereotypic response to cocaine was seen in these animals, which is in accord with the majority of reports showing no change or a decrease in dopamine receptor binding in the striatum following chronic stimulant administration (see Table 5.4B). Taken together, these data from nucleus accumbens and caudate nucleus injections indicate that there are no cocaine-induced alterations in dopamine receptor sensitivity sufficient to produce altered response to intracerebral stimulants.

Antelman and Chiodo (1981), Martres et al., 1977, and Schwartz et al. (1978) have suggested that stimulant-induced or dopamine agonist-induced behavioral sensitization might be due to autoreceptor desensitization. The dopamine autoreceptor is thought to exert inhibitory control over dopamine release and desensitization of this receptor would thus lead to an increased dopamine release and subsequent increased postsynaptic responsivity to a given pharmacological challenge. White and Wang (1984) have confirmed dopamine autoreceptor subsensitivity following chronic amphetamine in direct electrophysiological studies recording from single dopamine neurons of A10. Robinson and Becker (1982) reported that prior chronic administration of amphetamine led to an increased release of dopamine compared to saline-pretreated animals. These data are consistent with the hypothesis of dopamine autoreceptor desensitization, which would produce an increased presynaptic release of a neurotransmitter.

Low doses of apomorphine have been shown to decrease locomotor output in rodents (Carlsson, 1975). This paradoxical effect has been attributed to inhibition of dopaminergic neuronal activity induced by dopamine autoreceptor activation. To assess this possi-

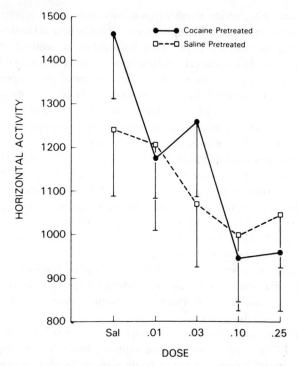

FIGURE 5.15. Lack of effect of chronic cocaine on low-dose apomorphine supression of activity. The group ($n=9$ or 10/group) mean horizontal activity for 30 minutes is plotted on the ordinate and the dose of apomorphine is plotted on the abscissa. The rats were pretreated for ten days with cocaine (10 mg/ml) or saline before being tested with one of several doses (0.0, 0.01, 0.03, 0.10, 0.25 mg/kg) of apomorphine, 24 hours following their last cocaine or saline injection. No differences in locomotor activity were observed between the cocaine- and saline-pretreated groups for any of these doses of apomorphine, suggesting that autoreceptor desensitization does not account for the increased behavioral effects of cocaine upon chronic administration.

bility, we challenged animals with a range of doses of apomorphine (0.01, 0.03, 0.10, 0.25 mg/kg, i.p.) one day following chronic cocaine (10 mg/kg) or saline administration for ten days. The results of this study suggest that dopamine autoreceptor sensitivity is not altered by this regimen of cocaine pretreatment (fig. 5.15).

Moreover, a study reported by Gale et al. (1981) raises the

possibility that dopaminergic mechanisms may not be critical to all types of cocaine-induced behavioral sensitization. They treated animals daily (for ten days) with high doses of cocaine (40 mg) subcutaneously, which were sufficient to produce (three days later) marked behavioral sensitization, that is, stereotypic sniffing and gnawing. These rats showed an increased response to cocaine (20 mg/kg i.p.), but a decreased response to apomorphine (0.4 mg/kg, s.c.). When animals were co-treated with a dopamine receptor blocking agent, the neuroleptic haloperidol (1.0 mg/kg, s.c.) which was sufficient to block cocaine-induced activation acutely, cocaine-treated animals still showed increased responsivity to cocaine (but not apomorphine) compared to saline pretreated animals. These data suggest that some nondopamine receptor components of cocaine's effects may be important to the induction of some types of sensitization. Beninger and Hahn (1983), however, reported that neuroleptic co-treatment would block the development but not the expression of sensitization induced by amphetamine (2.5 mg/kg, i.p.). We have also found that haloperidol (0.5 mg/kg) would block the development, but not the expression of sensitization induced by a single injection of cocaine (40 mg/kg). Diazepam (5 mg/kg) also blocked the sensitizing effects of cocaine (40 mg/kg), suggesting that expression of cocaine-induced behaviors (running and/or stereo-typy) *are* required for sensitization to occur to some types of cocaine pretreatment (i.e., lower dose or less chronic). The inability of neuroleptics to block the expression of stimulant-induced behavioral sensitization once it has been established may have important clinical implications. To the extent that stimulant-induced sensiti-zation is a useful model for the development of some types of psychosis, these observations could provide a basis for understanding neuroleptic nonresponsiveness clinically. This would particularly be the case where sensitization develops under conditions when neuroleptics are not initially employed and neuroleptics are subsequently used in an attempt to inhibit sensitization effects. Our data, and those of Beninger and Hahn (1983), suggest that while the development of sensitization is neuroleptic-responsive (and, presumably, dopamine-dependent), the manifestation or expression of behavioral sensitization is no longer dopamine-dependent, as revealed by the inability of high doses of neuroleptics to block the context-specific effects of prior cocaine. In this fashion, one might view the early use of neuroleptics as adequate for the prevention or "prophylaxis" of sensitization but inadequate to suppress or reverse the process one it have become manifest.

Gale et al. (1981) postulated that effects on gamma-amino-butyric acid (GABA) metabolism might be important to her type neuroleptic-independent sensitization, as chronic high-dose cocaine in their study led to 35% increases in glutamatic acid decarboxylase activity and a 40% decrease in GABA receptor binding in striatum, effects that were not blocked by haloperidol. Thiebot et al. (1981) reported enhancement of acute cocaine-induced hyperactivity by benzodiazepines (which could be blocked by picrotoxinin), further implicating GABAergic mechanisms. It is also possible that the local anaesthetic effects of cocaine are important to the behavioral sensitization.

In support of this argument, we have observed that repeated administration of subconvulsant doses of local anaesthetics lead to increasing effects on some behaviors, such as omniphagia (i.e., ingestion of inedible objects) (Post et al., 1976). The percentage of animals demonstrating this effect increases following repeated administration. Moreover, lidocaine-pretreated animals are subsequently more responsive to the behavioral-activating effects of cocaine (Squillace et al., 1982). These data are illustrated in Figure 5.16 and are important for several reasons. Since lidocaine is not a psychomotor stimulant and itself induces and sensitizes behaviors other than motor activity, the observed cross sensitization of lidocaine to cocaine suggests that the sensitization may be local anaesthetic-mediated, and is not merely an effect of conditioning.

These data are also consistent with the idea that conditioning cannot be the explanation for all aspects of stimulant-induced behavioral sensitization as a series of new behaviors appears to evolve on chronic administration. As emphasized by Ellinwood and Kilbey (1980) as well as Segal and Schuckit (1983), animals that initially show minor degrees of hyperactivity, upon repetition of stimulant administration show not just increasing degrees of locomotor behavior but the evolution of new and more bizarre and constricted behavioral sequences and stereotypies, and, ultimately, some aspects of dyskinetic behavior as well. Thus, this progressive evolution and unfolding of new behaviors in the sensitized repertoire are reminiscent of the process in electrical kindling where repeated stimulation of a given substrate not only produces increasingly widespread effects, but the behavioral and convulsive responsivity

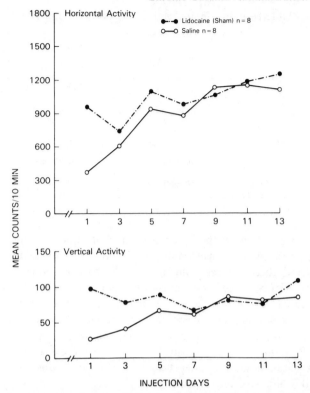

FIGURE 5.16. Cocaine-induced activity following lidocaine pretreatment. Lidocaine-pretreated animals demonstrated greater horizontal and vertical activity following the first cocaine injection than saline-pretreated controls ($p<.05$). This pretreatment difference diminished, however, as the saline group became more sensitized to the effects of cocaine. Activity was the mean counts/10 min for 90 minutes following the injection.

evolves with increasing complexity over time, until a full-blown major motor seizure is produced to a stimulus that had previously been ineffective (Table 5.1).

It is worthy of reemphasis, however, that the mechanisms underlying stimulant-induced behavioral sensitization may be very different from those responsible for producing convulsive endpoint achieved with either electrophysiological or pharmacological kindling. The evidence supporting differential mechanisms underlying behavioral sensitization and kindling are summarized in Table 5.5.

Table 5.5 Differences in Kindling and Behavioral Sensitization

	Electrical Kindling	Stimulant-induced Behavioral Sensitization
Measurement	Convulsive endpoint	Behavioral endpoint
Duration	Appears permanent	Long-lasting (wks-mos but decays)
Catecholamine potentiation	Inhibits	Facilitates
Stress	Inhibits	Facilitates
Vasopressin deficiency	Facilitates	Inhibits

While manipulations that increase catecholaminergic tone may potentiate behavioral sensitization, they tend to be anticonvulsant to amydala-kindled seizures. Similarly, while stress is shown to facilitate stimulant-induced sensitization in many instances, it has also been shown to retard the development of kindled seizures. In parallel, vasopressin definciency appears to retard cocaine-induced behavioral sensitization, yet may facilitate electrophysiological kindling (Putnam et al., unpublished data, 1983) and exert differential effects on rate of kindling, depending on anatomical substrate that is kindled (Gillis & Cain, 1983a,b).

These data are also consistent with the studies of Lesse (1980), Lesse and Collins (1980), and Stripling and Hendricks (1982) indicating that acute cocaine administration has complex effects on different aspects of the kindled seizure process. While cocaine may facilitate spread of electrical activity during the kindling process (Ellinwood et al., 1977) and lower afterdischarge thresholds in a frequency-dependent manner (Lesse & Collins, 1980; Stripling & Hendricks, 1983), it also decreases the afterdischarge duration. Again, these data may be interpretable on the basis of the dual effects of cocaine as both a local anaesthetic and potentiator of catecholamine systems. The former process may be associated with some seizure facilitation (Racine et al., 1975) while the latter may have anticonvulsant effects, as documented in many pharmacological dissections (see review of Peterson & Albertson, 1982).

These differential effects of cocaine may also explain why chronic cocaine, which appears to increase catecholamine mediated behavior, does not change or may retard subsequent amygdala kindling (Sato et al., 1980; Post et al., 1981b; Kilbey et al., 1979). However, when higher doses were administered (Kilbey et al., 1979) and cocaine-induced seizures produced, subsequent spread of electrical activity from amygdala to other areas of brain proceeded more rapidly. In addition, when seizures were induced by repeated administration of the pure local anaesthetic lidocaine, facilitation of subsequent electrical kindling of the amygdala was observed (Fig. 15.6).

The studies of Memo et al. (1981) and Hanbauer (p.c. 1983), as noted above, raise the possibility that alterations in cocaine binding or cocaine effects on cyclic-AMP and calcium calmodulin-stimulated adenylate cyclase in addition to effects on dopamine receptors (see Table 5.4A) could also be important to behavioral sensitization. These investigators reported that as early as 60 minutes after cocaine administration (20 mg/kg, i.p.), increases in [^{3}H]-spiroperidol and [^{3}H]-N-propylnorapomorphine were observed, as well as increases in membrane-bound calmodulin and responsiveness of adenylate cyclase to dopamine. Incubation of striatal slices with cocaine (10^{-6}M), but not with lidocaine (10^{-6}M) also produced receptor and cyclase changes.

The susceptibility of cocaine-induced behavioral sensitization to environmental context and conditioning elements raises the possibility that an environmentally responsive facilitatory pathway could impact on dopamine or other cocaine-mediated behaviors in a fashion parallel to that seen in the sensitization model in Aplysia. Kandel and co-workers (1982) have described sensitization of the gill withdrawal reflex in Aplysia based on prior conditioning. This involves potentiation of neurotransmission at a serotonergic synapse, presumably by presynaptic facilitation. Aspects of the molecular mechanisms of this response have been described in detail and are thought to involve long-term changes in biochemical responsivity involving cyclic-AMP, calcium channel fluxes, as well as, ultimately, the structure of the involved synapse. Whether such a mechanism is involved in the processes underlying cocaine-induced behavioral sensitization remains to be elucidated, but is an interesting possibility. Similarly, the possible parallels or differences between cocaine-induced behavioral and convulsive sensitivity changes and other models involving long-term synaptic responsivity based on prior stimulation, such as that involved in long-term potentiation and kindling, are an important area of investigation.

The elucidation of the important mechanisms involved in cocaine sensitization and kindling may ultimately prove of clinical import in treating long-term behavioral changes that may be occurring in humans following chronic cocaine administration. The direct relevance of cocaine-induced behavioral syndromes in animals to the signs and symptoms observed in humans remains to be established. However, many factors that modulate cocaine-induced behavioral sensitization and toxicity in animals may be applicable to phenomena occuring in humans and deserve to be examined on the basis of available, but indirect, epidemiological data or directly tested in the context of controlled clinical research designs.

ACUTE AND CHRONIC EFFECTS OF COCAINE IN HUMANS

The mood-elevating and psychomotor stimulant effects of cocaine have been known for centuries. Descriptions of the effects of early use of cocaine have been provided elsewhere (Byck, 1975; Post, 1976; Peterson, 1977; Siegel, 1977, 1984) but one sociological phenomenon perhaps deserves emphasis here. Assessment of the potential dangers and toxicity of cocaine appears to undergo cyclic variation. After Freud and others became enamored of cocaine's positive effects on mood and behavior, Freud became increasingly convinced of its potential liabilities. Eventually cocaine was called "the third scourge of mankind."

Following this period of acknowledgment and, perhaps, overemphasis of cocaine's behaviorally and physiologically toxic properties, these data appeared to be largely ignored and cocaine, particularly in the last several decades, emerged as king and queen of the drug realm, the "Gift of the Sun God" (Gay et al., 1973), the quintessential drug of abuse capable of producing exquisite highs purportedly without addiction. Cocaine was even casually described in some public forums as "as safe as chicken soup."

> "Cocaine is less harmful than many other legal and illegal drugs popular in America. Most of the evidence is that there aren't any adverse effects to normal cocaine use. It looks to be much safer than barbiturates and amphetamines, and there's no evidence it has the body effects of cigarettes or alcohol. If I were going to go out and sell a drug to the public, it would probably be cocaine. We might be better off using it as a recreational drug than marihuana. (*San Francisco Chronicle*, Thursday, October 21, 1976, p. 4 quoted in Wesson & Smith, 1977)

There appears no good reason and even less evidence to suggest that cocaine is an especially dangerous drug. The large single doses given for medical reasons have at times produced extremely serious toxic reactions, the doses used in social settings have not. At any rate a search of the relevant literature fails to show a single case of serious toxic reaction in the past forty years or so.

The conclusion that cocaine is not a dangerous pleasure drug is buttressed by the fact that pure cocaine, when taken in the normal social doses of 20–30 mg repeated every 30 to 60 min., and administered in the most common way—by snorting—is not the extremely potent drug it has been made out to be. (in *Cocaine, Its History, Uses and Effects* by Richard Ashley, Warner Books, N.Y., 1975)

Appropriate recognition of its dangers now appears to be again in vogue. Finkle and McCloskey (1977) described 111 deaths involving cocaine; 86 were drug-related (60 involved drug combinations, 26 involved cocaine alone). One-third of the victims died in the first hour, apparently by "seizures followed by respiratory arrest."

In spite of Ashley and other's claims to the contrary, there was mounting evidence of cocaine's involvement in sudden, unexplained death as a function of year.

1971	1972	1973	1974	1975	1976
2	3	11	25	37	58*

(*extrapolated from Finkle & McCloskey, 1977)

By 1983–84, cocaine-related problems were epidemic and a toll-free 800-COCAINE number received 300,000 calls (70,000 in the first twelve weeks and currently as many as 1000 calls/day), revealing a variety of psychological and physiological effects of the social use of cocaine (Washton & Gold, 1984).

With cocaine use becoming increasingly widespread (it is estimated that as many as thirty million people in the United States have experimented with the drug), psychological and physiological problems are becoming apparent. In the surveys of Siegel (1977, 1984) and that of Washton and Gold (1984) using a toll-free number and assessing the reports of the first 500 self-referred cocaine users, a fairly consistent picture is emerging. Dysphoric moods, paranoid trends, and full-blown paranoid episodes are being reported subjectively as well as increasingly observed in emergency room settings. A moderate incidence of cocaine-induced seizures or

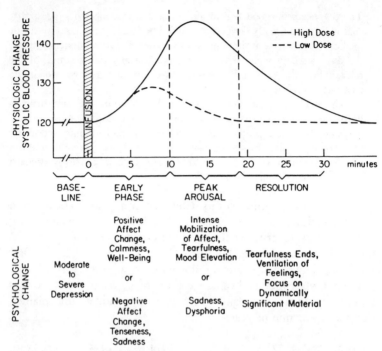

FIGURE 5.17. Effects of intravenous cocaine on mood and physiology in depressed patients

blackouts (17%) is also being reported in these surveys. One must be conservative in the interpretation of these data based on the largely unknown doses and compositions of substances being ingested. Yet, the similarity of these reports to those observed under more controlled conditions and to some of the behaviors and physiological effects produced in the animal laboratories (i.e., sensitization to seizures) remain striking.

When we administered cocaine intravenously to depressed patients, we did not find a substantial antidepressant effect. While some patients reported mood elevation, particularly with lower doses associated with mild to moderate alterations in pulse and blood pressure (Fig. 5.17), doses that were associated with more marked physiological activation often produced a mixed or dysphoric picture. Many patients showed a syndrome of tearful reminiscence; some patients appreciated the situation as subjectively positive, but others found it extremely dysphoric. In some instances, there was a marked subjective-objective dissociation. The experimenter might see an anguished facial expression in the subject who reported, while tearful, that he never felt better in his life (Post et al., 1974). This dissociation is also noteworthy in light of the reports by Adamec and associates (p.c. 1983) that a similar objective-subjective dissociation could be observed in some subjects receiving the pure local anaesthetic procaine.

Based on electrophysiological and deoxyglucose studies which suggested that procaine appeared to exert some relative selectivity for activating limbic system substrates, we thought that it might prove to be a useful probe of limbic system sensitivity and dysfunction among patients with hypothesized limbic system dysfunction. We were encouraged by the reports of Kenneth Livingston (personal communication) who had utilized intravenous procaine in the treatment of patients with a variety of behavioral and pain syndromes with great safety. We adopted the paradigm that he developed in collaboration with R. Adamec and C. Adamec of giving increasing intravenous doses of procaine preceded by and interspersed with saline placebo administration (Adamec et al., 1985) in order to assess behavioral, physiological, electrophysiological, cognitive, and endocrine effects of this agent. The maximum dose of procaine utilized was 2.3 mg/kg i.p., a dose well below that which would be convulsant. A series of five increasing doses with this as the maximum dose were employed in each patient receiving a "long" procedure involving three placebo administrations. Following experience with this paradigm, a shorter version was employed utilizing an initial placebo administration and the first and fourth doses of procaine (0.46 mg/kg and 1.84 mg/kg, respectively) that were used in the long procedure.

To date, the data on seven affectively ill patients, seventeen patients with borderline personality disorders, and seven normal volunteer controls have been analyzed (Kellner et all, 1986). Intravenous procaine was associated with dose-related increases in disturbances in sensory and cognitive functioning. Tinnitus was reported with increasing frequency and intensity as a function of dose. In addition, patients reported increased auditory acuity and a variety of distortions of visual and auditory modalities, and two patients reported smelling tuna fish. Two patients also recalled affectively charged reminiscences with such a vividness of imagery and immediacy of experiential phenomena that they resembled hallucinatory episodes, yet were clearly differentiated by the patient

Table 5.6 Effects of Cocaine Potentially Related to its Local Anaesthetic Properties

---

Acute effects
  Mood lability (euphoria)
  Anxiety-dysphoria
  Tinnitus
  Sensory distortions
  Hallucinatory-like phenomena
  Seizures
  Cardio-respiratory arrest

Chronic effects
  Sensitization to bizarre behaviors
  Seizure sensitization (kindling)
  Interictal irritability and aggression
  Panic attacks?

---

from an hallucinatory experience. These cognitive and sensory effects were associated with a wide variety of mood alterations ranging from several patients experiencing mood elevation and euphoria to extreme dysphoria and near panic. Dysphoric responses were more prominent in patients with borderline personality disturbances than either affectively ill patients or normal volunteer controls, although these differences may reflect baseline differences. Increases in fast EEG frequencies were observed selectively of the temporal cortex (Coppola et al., 1983; unpublished manuscript 1984), further supporting data in animals that local anesthetics may exert some selectivity for the temporal lobe and limbic substrates (Wagman et al., 1967). The degree of psychosensory distortion and dysphoria was significantly correlated with the degree of EEG activation in temporal cortical areas. In the group as a whole, dose-related increases in prolactin secretion were observed while there was no significant effect on growth hormone. ACTH and cortisol were stimulated by procaine in an apparent dose-related fashion. It is noteworthy that stimulation of ACTH and cortisol occurred independently of whether patients reported subjective euphoric or dysphoric experiences, suggesting the possibility that procaine might have direct effects (independent of the degree of distress) in stimulating the hypothalamic-pituitary-adrenal axis, potentially by directly releasing CRF. Preliminary evidence for this phenomenon comes from the studies of Gold, Gallucci, Kling, and associates (unpublished observation, 1985) in sheep subjected to ventricular cannulization. In these animals, procaine administration led to the release of CRF into the ventricular CSF, but not into plasma, while ACTH increased in plasma, but not CSF.

The clinical data with the pure local anaesthetic, procaine, in three different subject populations suggest that some components of the cocaine syndrome may be mediated by cocaine's potent local anaesthetic properties (Table 5.6). These might include the experience of sensory and cognitive alterations and hallucinatory-like phenomena in all sensory modalities (Siegel, 1977), intensification of sounds and ringing in the ears (Siegel, 1984), and anxiety, irritability, and aggression. Sixty-six percent of cocaine hotline callers (Washton & Gold, 1984) reported fighting and violent arguments, findings also of interest in relation to the aggressive behavior in rats (Post, 1981a; Post et al., 1984) seen after local anaesthetic (lidocaine) seizures.

Although most patients in our infusion study found the procaine experience neutral to subjectively unpleasant, several subjects who had no prior experience with stimulants did report mood elevation. Van Dyke and associates (1979) also reported that lidocaine administered to experienced cocaine users produced self-reported mood elevation not distinguishable from that associated with their habitual use of cocaine. However, a conditioned affective response to the local anaesthetic properties cannot be ruled out in this instance. The major component of cocaine's euphoriant properties is probably related to its psychomotor stiumlant properties, since other stimulants, such as amphetamine and methylphenidate, which are not potent local anaesthetics, share cocaine's ability to markedly potentiate catecholamines, and also produce parallel effects on mood (Martin et al., 1971; Ellinwood & Kilbey, 1977; Fischman et al., 1976). Fischman (1984) described differential effects of procaine vs. lidocaine compared to cocaine in volunteers. Subjects identified 48 and 96 mg of procaine as cocaine, but all doses of lidocaine and 16 and 32 mg of procaine were identified as placebo. Procaine, but not lidocaine, has also been reported to support self-administration in experimental animals (Ford & Balster, 1977; Woolverton & Balster, 1979).

Discriminative stimulus studies also document the dual properties of cocaine (Colpaert et al., 1978; 1979). Dopaminergic mechanisms appear to be involved in cocaine's discriminative stimulus properties since low doses of cocaine generalize to amphetamine and methylphenidate, and cocaine's effects are blocked by neuroleptics.

However, higher doses of cocaine (20 mg/kg) (Shearman & Lal, 1981) generalized to the discriminative stimulus properties of pentylenetetrazol (20 mg/kg), which is anxiogenic and convulsant. Aston-Jones et al. (1984) also reported that cocaine blocked the anxiolytic effects of alcohol, further suggesting an anxiogenic effect of cocaine. Diazepam (but not haloperidol) antagonized the discriminative stimulus properties of pentylenetetrazol or cocaine (20 mg/kg) (Shearman & Lal, 1981). These data are consistent with our observations in depressed patients (Post et al., 1974) and those in the literature that low doses of cocaine are likely to be euphorogenic and non-anxiogenic, while higher doses (which do not generalize to the lower in discriminative stimulus studies) may be anxiogenic (Siegel et al., 1984; Grinspoon & Bakalar, 1976; Resnick, 1977), possibly on the basis of the local anaesthetic component of cocaine. Anxiety and dysphoric effects may increasingly predominate if tolerance develops to the euphorogenic effects of cocaine, as frequently reported, and doses of cocaine are rapidly escalated in an attempt to maintain the peak mood elevation.

The dysphoria, fear, and, in rare instances, near panic produced by procaine would suggest that these local anaesthetic effects could be the substrate for similar effects reported with cocaine. Intense anxiety associated with cocaine use has long been noted and is the often cited reason for attempting to modulate this process with the use of associated drugs such as heroin, commonly referred to as "speed balling." Washton and Gold (1984) also reported that 60% of their cocaine hotline callers were using alcohol or sedative or hypnotic drugs to reduce the "jittery" stimulant effects of cocaine or to relieve the wearoff crash. If anxiety and dysphoria to cocaine showed sensitization or kindling-like effects similar to those observed in our animal laboratory studies, it could provide an explanation for the mounting anxiety, irritability, and dysphoria reported with more chronic administration in some, particularly high-dose and compulsive, cocaine users (Siegel, 1984).

It is noteworthy in the studies of Washton and Tatarsky (1984) and Washton and Gold (1984) that a 20 to 50% incidence of panic attacks has been reported in these self-referred abusers of cocaine. T. W. Uhde, M. Geraci, B. Vittone, P. Roy-Byrne and associates, studying patients with panic anxiety disorders, have observed a series of patients who reported experiencing their first panic attacks following cocaine ingestion. An example of such a patient is illustrated in Figure 5.18 (Uhde et al., unpublished observations). This patient reported essentially daily cocaine administration for several years prior to the onset of his first panic attack, which occurred immediately following the ingestion of cocaine by the nasal route. He subsequently had a series of cocaine-induced panic attacks which always immediately followed cocaine administration. However, many ingestions were not associated with such a panic attack. Following many repetitions of cocaine-related panic attacks, the patient had his first spontaneous or non-cocaine-related panic episode, which led to the progressive development of agoraphobia and increased generalized anxiety symptoms. At this point, the patient discontinued cocaine use, since he surmised that the cocaine had also been etiologic in the development of the spontaneous panic attacks. [These "spontaneous" panic attacks subsequently responded moderately well to alprazolam, exacerbated during its withdrawal, and also responded well to carbamazepine and to imipramine (Uhde et al., 1984).]

This patient's course is of considerable interest in relation to a possible sensitization or kindling-like mechanism. Did repeated cocaine use in this patient lead to a kindling-like lowering of the threshold for and an increased incidence of cocaine-induced panic reactions that then went on to a "spontaneous" phase, occurring in the absence of cocaine administration? It is of interest that many repetitions of amygdala-kindled seizures are required (often hundreds of stimulations in the rat) before spontaneous seizures are observed (Post et al., 1981b). Our data in repeated local anaesthetic administration to animals would suggest that it is possible that the local anaesthetic effects of cocaine in themselves could produce a kindling-like mechanism (Post et al., 1975; 1984). Moreover, we have observed several animals given repeated lidocaine-induced seizures go on to a spontaneous phase (like that observed following repeated kindled seizures) where they had developed seizures in the absence of lidocaine administration (Contel & Post, unpublished observations). Data that animals will self-administer cocaine to the point of convulsions and death (Deneau et al., 1969; Johanson, 1984) may also be comprehensible from either a kindled-seizure or total dose lethality perspective.

Clearly, further work is required in order to establish a direct link between behavioral sensitization and kindling-like mechanisms and various psychological and physiological consequences of cocaine use in humans in uncontrolled clinical settings. However, utilization of these models may suggest specific strategies for testing this hypoth-

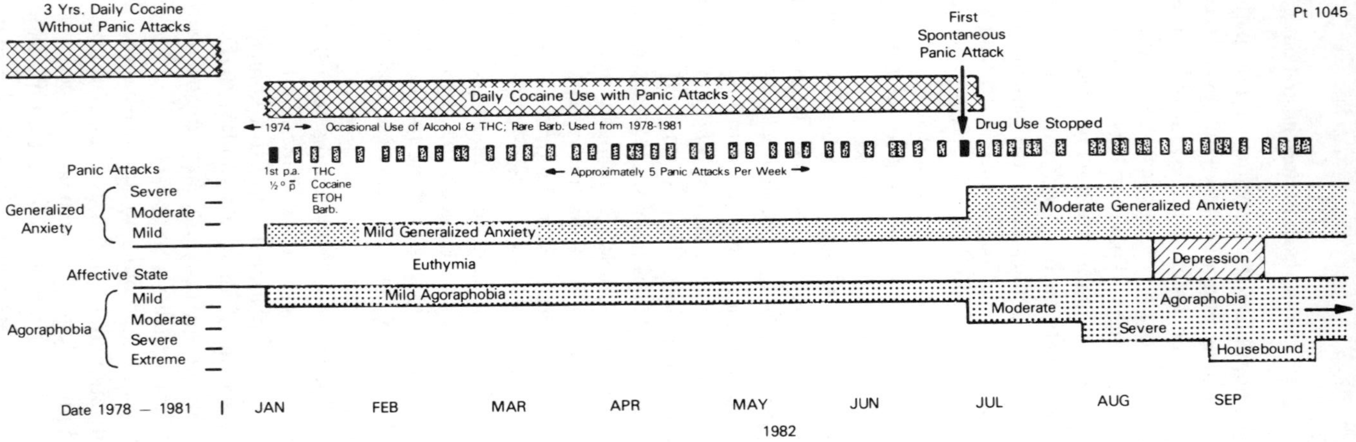

FIGURE 5.18 Development of panic disorder following cocaine use. The course of development of panic disorder for an individual patient, who used cocaine, is illustrated. Following three years of cocaine use, essentially daily by the intranasal route, this patient began to develop panic attacks immediately after cocaine use. Panic attacks occurred approximately three times/week for the next 6 months. Following these many repetitions of cocaine-induced panic attacks, he developed the first spontaneous panic attack, at which time the patient discontinued his cocaine use and developed more severe psychiatric symptoms, that is, generalized anxiety and agoraphobia.

158

esis and developing potential treatment approaches. Preliminary evidence (Post et al., 1984b) suggests that lithium, but not carbamazepine, may be effective in inhibiting cocaine-induced behavioral sensitization. Moreover, seizures have been reported as a consequence of cocaine and related local anaesthetic administration in humans, such that assessment of this endpoint, which is more directly parallel to that used in the animal models, may allow even better testing of the kindling hypothesis. Based on diazepam's ability to inhibit lidocaine-induced seizure sensitization (Fig. 5.4), one would postulate that it might be effective in preventing cocaine-induced seizure sensitization; neuroleptics might also help with dopaminergic aspects of toxicity (Jones, 1984), but would likely be ineffective against symptoms relating to behavioral sensitization (Gale et al., 1981). We have observed that carbamazepine is highly effective in inhibiting the development of lidocaine-kindled seizures produced by repeated administration of lidocaine (65 mg/kg, i.p.), but is ineffective in suppressing these seizures once they are fully manifest (Weiss, Szele, & Post, in preparation). In a parallel fashion, carbamaze- partially inhibits the development of cocaine-induced seizures and lethality, but is ineffective and may even enhance seizures and lethality to high doses of cocaine (Weiss, Woodward, & Post, unpublished data).

If the kindling hypothesis were borne out clinically, it would also have obvious implications for warnings regarding drug usage. Repeated administration of a given dose of cocaine without resulting seizures would in no way assure the continued safety of this drug even for that given individual and even assuming equal purity of the drug used. It is possible that some apparent "idiosyncratic" psychological and physiological crisis reactions to cocaine might be explainable from this kindling perspective.

We have also observed another problematic side effect that has been anecdotally associated with cocaine administration—dysphoric activation and psychosis (Post, 1975). As illustrated in Figure 5.19, following an unsuccessful antidepressant trial of oral cocaine in a moderately depressed inpatient, intravenous cocaine was administered in an attempt at more effective antidepressant therapy. Instead of an antidepressant response, the patient showed a marked deterioration in the severity of his depression with associated development of psychotic components. These observations may parallel the experience in some cocaine users who develop paranoia (self-

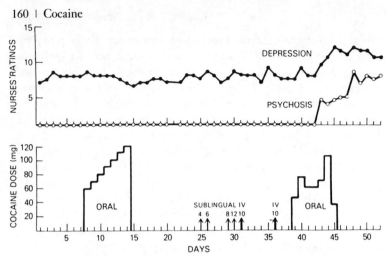

FIGURE 5.19. Sudden emergence of psychotic depression following inter-mittent cocaine administration. This figure illustrates the course of illness of a patient who was chronically depressed and given cocaine in an attempt to alleviate the depression (Post et al., 1974). Following some suggestion of a weak antidepressant response to oral cocaine, other routes of administration (sublingual and intravenous) were employed in an attempt to achieve more adequate absorption and blood levels. During a second trial of oral cocaine, the patient developed a marked exacerbation of his depression, which included a paranoid and psychotic component. In retrospect, these multiple attempts at achieving a euphoriant effect of cocaine may have inadvertently produced an adverse behavioral sensitization effect.

reported as 65% in the series of Washton & Gold, 1984) and psychosis (Siegel et al., 1984).

Again, we might ask the question whether phenomena and mechanisms akin to those documented in behavioral sensitization in animals (Figs. 5.7–5.12) are also involved in these clinical situations in humans. Many of the "known" relatively late effects of repeated cocaine administration in humans (including dysphoria, paranoid psychosis, mounting anxiety and panic attacks, and seizures) are not inconsistent with either a behavioral sensitization (Fig. 5.20) or kindling perspective. Systematic study of these phenomena may provide a comprehensible framework for further testing the clinical applicability of these models, their predictive validity, and possible new directions for clinical intervention.

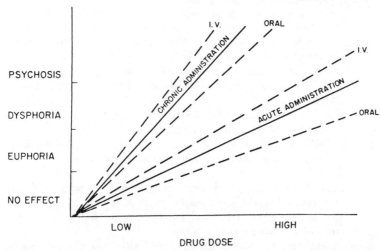

FIGURE 5.20. Interaction of dose, duration, and route of administration on cocaine-induced psychopathology. This schematic figure illustrates the hypothetical effects of cocaine following chronic or acute administration by various routes at various doses. Based on clinical and laboratory studies in the literature, it appears that less desirable effects of cocaine become more apparent after chronic administration and begin to appear following lower doses than with acute administration. Intravenous (or inhalation) administration may produce more psychopathological symptoms (Washton & Gold, 1984) than oral administration, because of more rapid absorption and higher blood levels.

REFERENCES

Adamec R., Stark-Adamec, C., Saint-Hilaire, J., Livingston, K. (1985) Basic science and clinical aspects of procaine HCl as a limbic system excitant. *Prog. Neuropsychopharmacol. Biol. Psychiat. 9:109–119.*

Akiyama, K., Sato, M., Kashihara, K., Otsuki, S. (1982a) Lasting changes in high affinity ^{3}H-spiperone binding to the rat striatum and mesolimbic area after chronic methamphetamine administration: evaluation of dopaminergic and serotonergic receptor components. *Biol. Psychiat.* 17:1389–1402.

Akiyama, K., Sato, M., Otsuki, S. (1982b) Increased ^{3}H-spiperone binding sites in mesolimbic area related to methamphetamine-induced behavioral hypersensitivity. *Biol. Psychiat.* 17:223–231.

Algeri, S., Brunello, N., Vantini, G. (1980) Different adaptive responses by rat striatal dopamine synthetic and receptor mechanisms after

162 | Cocaine

repeated treatment with d-amphetamine, methylphenidate and nomifensine. *Pharmacol. Res. Commun.* 12:675–681.

Antelman, S.M., Chiodo, L.A. (1981) Dopamine autoreceptor subsensitivy: a mechanism common to the treatment of depression and the indication of amphetamine psychosis. *Biol. Psychiat.* 16:717–727.

Ashley, R. (1975) Cocaine: its history, uses and effects. New York: Warner Books.

Aston-Jones, S., Aston-Jones, G., Koob, G.F. (1984) Cocaine antagonizes anxiolytic effects of ethanol. *Psychopharmol.* 84:28–31.

Banerjee, S.P., Sharma, V.K., Kung, L.S., Chanda, S.K. (1978) Amphetamine induces beta-adrenergic receptor supersensitivy. *Nature* 271:380–381.

Banerjee, S.P., Sharma, V.K., Kung-Cheung, L.S., Chanda, S.K., Riggi, S.J. (1979) Cocaine and d-amphetamine induce changes in central beta-adrenoceptor sensitivity: effects of acute and chronic drug treatment. *Brain Res.* 175:119–130.

Baudry, M., Martres, M.P., Schwartz, J.C. (1977) *In vivo* binding of ³H-pimozide in mouse striatum: effects of dopamine agonists and antagonists. *Life Sci.* 21:1163–1170.

Beninger, R.J., Hahn, B.L. (1983) Pimozide blocks establishment but not expression of amphetamine-produced environment-specific conditioning. *Science* 220:1304–1306.

Borison, R.L., Hitri, A., Klawans, H.L., Diamond, B.I. (1979) A new animal model for schizophrenia: behavioral and receptor binding studies. In Usdin, E., Kopin, I.J., Barchas, J. (eds.), *Catecholamines: Basic and Clinical Frontiers.* New York: pergamon Press, pp. 719–721.

Burt, D.R., Creese, I., Synder, S.H. (1977) Antischizophrenic drugs: chronic treatment elevated dopamine receptor binding in brain. *Science* 197:326–328.

Byck, R. (ed.) (1975) *Cocaine papers: Sigmund Freud.* New York: Stonehill Publishing Co.

Carlsson, A. (1975) Receptor-mediated control of dopamine metabolism. In Usdin, E., Bunney, W.E. Jr. (eds.), *Pre- and Postsynaptic Receptors.* New York: Marcel Dekker, pp. 49–66.

Chanda, S.K., Sharma, V.K., Banerjee, S.P. (1979) Beta-Adrenoceptor (B-AR) sensitivity following psychotropic drug treatment. In Usdin, E., Kopin, I.J., Barchas, J. (eds.) *Catecholamines: Basic and Clinical Frontiers.* New York: Pergamon Press, pp. 586–588.

Collins, J.P., Lesse, H., Dagan, L.W. (1979) Behavioral antecedents of cocaine-induced stereotypy. *Pharmacol. Biochem. Behav.* 11:683–687.

Colpaert, F.C., Niemegeers, C.J.E., Janssen, P.A.J. (1976) Cocaine cue in rats as it relates to subjective drug effects: a preliminary report. *Eur. J. Pharmacol.* 40:195–199.

Colpaert, F.C., Niemegeers, C.J.E., Janssen, P.A.J. (1978) Discriminative stimulus properties of cocaine and d-amphetamine and antagonism by haloperidol: a comparative study. *Neuropharmacol.* 17:937–942.

Colpaert, F.C., Niemegeers, C.J., Janssen, P.A. (1979) Discriminative stimulus properties of cocaine: neuropharmacological characteristics as derived from stimulus generalization experiments. *Pharmacol. Biochem. Behav.* 10:535–546.

Coppola, R., Salb, J., Chassey, J. 1983) Topographic analysis of epileptiform discharges. *Abstracts of the 15th Epilepsy International Symposium*, Washington D.C., September 26–30, 1983, p. 474.

Creese, I., Iversen, S.D. (1974) The role of forebrain dopamine systems in amphetamine-induced sterotypy in the adult rat following neonatal treatment with 6-hydroxydopamine. *Psychopharmacol.* 39:345–357.

Deneau, G.A., Yanagita, T., Seevers, M.H. (1969) Self administration of psychoactive substances by the monkey. *Psychopharmacol.* 16:30–48.

Downs, A.W., Eddy, N.B. (1932a) The effect of repeated doses of cocaine on the dog. *J. Pharmacol. Exp. Ther.* 46:195.

Downs, A.W., Eddy, N.B. (1932b) The effect of repeated doses of cocaine on the rat. *J. Pharmacol. Exp. Ther.* 46:199.

Eichler, A.J., Antelman, S.M., Black, C.A. (1980) Amphetamine sterotypy is not a homogeneous phenomenon: sniffing and licking show distinct profiles of sensitization and tolerance. *Psychopharmacol.* 68:287–290.

Ellinwood, E.H., Kilbey, M.M. (1975) Amphetamine stereotypy: the influence of environmental factors and prepotent behavioral patterns on its topography and development. *Biol. Psychiat.* 10:3–16.

Ellinwood, E.H., Kilbey, M.M. (1980) Fundamental mechanisms underlying altered behavior following chronic administration of psychomotor stimulants. *Biol. Psychiat.* 15:749–757.

Ellinwood, E.H., Kilbey, M.M., Castellani, S., Khoury, C. (1977) Amygdala hyperspindling and seizures induced by cocaine. In Ellinwood, E.H., Kilbey, M.M. (eds.) *Advances in Behavioral Biology*, Vol. 21, *Cocaine and Other Stimulants*. New York: Plenum, pp. 303–326.

Finkle, B.S., McCloskey, K.L. (1977) The forensic toxicology of cocaine. In Petersen, R.C., Stillman, R.C. (eds.), *Cocaine: 1977*. NIDA Research Monograph No. 13. Washington D.C.: U.S. Government Printing Office, pp. 153–192.

Fischman, M.W. (1984) The behavioral pharmacology of cocaine in humans. In Grabowski, J. (ed.), *Cocaine: Pharmacology, Effects and*

Treatment of Abuse. NIDA Research Monograph No. 50 Washington, D.C.: U.S. Government Printing Office, pp. 72–91.

Fischman, M.W., Schuster, C.R., Krasnegor, N. (1977) Physiological and behavioral effects of intravenous cocaine in man. In Ellinwood, E.H., Kilbey, M.M. (eds.), *Advances in Behavioral Biology*, Vo. 21, *Cocaine and Other Stimulants.* New York: Plenum, pp. 647–664.

Fischman, M.W., Schuster, C.R., Resnikov, L., Shick, J.F.E., Krasnegor, N.A., Fennell, W., Freedman, D.X. (1976) Cardiovascular and subjective effects of intravenous cocaine administration in humans. *Arch. Gen. Psychiat.* 33:983–989.

Ford, R.D., Balster, R.L. (1977) Reinforcing properties of intravenous procaine in rhesus monkeys. *Pharmacol. Biochem. Behav.* 6:289–296.

Friedhoff, A.J., Bonnet, K., Rosengarten, H. (1977) Reversal of two manifestations of dopamine receptor supersensitivity by administration of L-DOPA. *Res. Commun. Chem. Pathol. Pharmacol.* 16:411–423.

Gale, K., Marshall, D., Bernstein, H., Butler, J. (1981) Effects of chronic cocaine administration on nigrostriatal function: neurochemical and behavioral changes in rats (Abstr No. 325). *Fed. Proc. 40: 291.*

Gay, G.R., Sheppard, C.W., Inaba, D.S., Newmeyer, J.A. (1973) Cocaine in perspective: "Gift from the Sun God" to "The Rich Man's Drug." *Drug Forum* 2:409–430.

Gillis, B.J., Cain, D.P. (1983a) Amygdala and pyriform cortex kindling in vasopressin deficient rats. *Brain Res.* 271:375–378.

Gillis, B.J., Cain, D.P. (1983b) Fascilitation of electrical kindling in ventral hippocampus and lateral septum in vasopressin deficient rats. *Abstracts of the Society for Neuroscience*, 13th Annual Mtg, Boston November 6–11, 1983, Abstr. No. 144.4, p. 484.

Globus, M., Bannet, J., Lerer, B., Belmaker, R.H. (1982) The effect of chronic bromocriptine and L-Dopa on spiperone binding and apomorphine-induced stereotypy. *Psychopharmacol.* 78:81–84.

Goddard, G.V., McIntyre, D.C., Leech, C.K. (1969) A permanent change in brain function resulting from daily electrical stimulation. Exp. Neurol. 25:295–330.

Goeders, N.E., Smith, J.E. (1983) Cortical dopaminergic involvement in cocaine reinforcement. *Science* 221:773–775.

Goeders, N.E., Smith, J.E. (1984) Effects of 6-hydroxydopamine lesions of the medial prefrontal cortex on intracranial cocaine self-administration. *Soc. for Neuroscience Abstracts*, Vol. 10, 14th Annual Meeting, Anaheim, Calif., October 10–15, 1984, Abstr. No. 347.5, p. 1206.

Grinspoon, L., Bakalar, J.B. (1976) *Cocaine: A Drug and its Social Evolution.* New York: Basic Books.

Gutierrez-Noriega, C. (1950) Inhibition of central nervous systems produced by chronic cocaine intoxication. *Fed. Proc.* 9:280.

Gutierrez-Noriega, C., Zapata-Oriz, V. (1944) Cocainismo experimental. Toxicologia general acostumbramiento y sensibilizacion. *Rev. Med. Exp.* (Lima) 3:297.

Hadfield, M.G., Nugent, E.A. (1985) Cocaine: comparative effect on dopamine uptake in extrapyramidal and limbic systems. *Biochem. Pharmacol.* 15: 744–746.

Hanbauer, I., Memo, M., Pradhan, S. (1981) Injection of cocaine causes supersensitivity of adenylate cyclase-coupled dopamine receptors and an increase of calmodulin content in rat striatal membrane fractions. *Proceedings of Society for Neurochemistry*, 1981.

Hertting, G., Axelrod, J., Kopin, I.J., Whitby, L.G. (1961) Lack of uptake of catecholamines after chronic denervation of sympathetic nerves. *Nature* 189:66.

Hinson, R.E., Poulos, C.X. (1981) Sensitization to the behavioral effects of cocaine: modification by Pavlovian conditioning. *Pharmacol. Biochem. Behav.* 15:559–562.

Hitri, A., Klawans, H.L. (1978) d-Amphetamine and levodopa induced changes in striatal membrane dopamine binding. *Proceedings 11th CINP Congress*, July 9–14, 1978, p. 90.

Hitzemann, R.J., Wu, J., Hom, D., Loh, H.H. (1980) Brain locations controlling the behavioral effects of chronic amphetamine intoxication. *Psychopharmacol.* 72:93–101.

Howlett, D.R., Nahorski, S.R. (1978) Effect of acute and chronic amphetamine administration on beta-adrenoceptors and dopamine receptors in rat corpus striatum and limbic forebrain. *Br. J. Pharmacol.* 64:411P–412P.

Isaac, W., Neiswander, J., Landers, T., Alcala, R., Bardo, M., Nonnerman, A. (1984) Mesocortical dopamine system lesions disrupt cocaine reinforced conditioned place preference. *Society for Neuroscience Abstracts*, Vol. 10. 14th Annual Meeting, Anaheim, Calif., October 10–15, 1984, Abstr. 7 No. 347.6, p. 1206.

Jackson, D.M., Baily, R.C., Christie, M.S., Crisp, E.A., Skerritt, J.H. (1981) Long-term d-amphetamine in rats: lack of change in post-synaptic dopamine receptor sensitivity. *Psychopharmacol.* 73:276–280.

Jackson, D.M., Jenkins, O.F., Malor, R., Christie, M.J., Gregory, P. (1983) Chronic L-Dopa treatment of rats and mice does not change the sensitivity of post-synaptic dopamine receptors. *Neunyn-Schmiedebergs Arch. Pharmacol.* 324:271–274.

Johanson, C.E. (1984) Assessment of the dependence potential of cocaine in animals. In Grabowski, J. (ed.), *Cocaine: Pharmacology, Effects, and*

Treatment of Abuse. NIDA Research Monograph No. 50, Washington, D.C.: U.S. Government Printing Office, pp. 72–91.

Jones, R.T. (1984) The Pharmacology of Cocaine. In Grabowski, J. (ed.), *Cocaine: Pharmacology, Effects, and Treatment of Abuse.* NIDA Research Monograph No. 50. Washington, D.C.: U.S. Government Printing Office, pp. 34–53.

Kandel, E.R., Schwartz, J.H. (1982) Molecular biology of learning: modulation of transmitter release. *Science* 218:433–443.

Kelley, P.H., Iversen, S.D. (1975) Selective 6-OHDA-induced destruction of mesolimbic dopamine neurons: abolition of psychostimulant-induced locomotor activity in rats. *Eur. J. Pharmacol.* 40:45–56.

Kellner C.H. Post, R.M., Putnam, F. Cowdry, R., Gardner, D., Kling, M.A., Minichiello, M.A, and Coppola, R. (1986) Intravenous procaine as a probe of limbic system activity in psychiatric patients and normal controls. *Biol. Psychiat.* (in press).

Kennedy, L.T., Hanbauer, I. (1982) ^{3}H-Cocaine binding in rat brain: modulation by Na+ and an endogenous inhibitor. *Fed. Proc.* 41:1328.

Kilbey, M.M., Ellinwood, E.H., Easler, M.E. (1979) The effects of chronic cocaine pretreatment on kindled seizures and behavioral stereotypies. *Exp. Neurol.* 64:306–314.

Klawans, H.L., Goetz, C., Nausieda, P.A., Weiner, W.J. (1977a) Levodopa-induced dopamine receptor hypersensitivity. *Ann. Neurol.* 2:125–129.

Klawans, H.L., Hitri, A., Carvey, P.M., Nausieda, P.A., Weiner, W.J. (1979a) Effect of chronic dopaminergic agonism on striatal membrane dopamine binding. In Poirier, L.J., Sourkes, T.L., Bedard, P.J. (eds.) *Advances in Neurology*, Vol. 24. New York: Raven Press, pp. 217–224.

Klawans, H.L., Hitri, A., Nausieda, P.A., Weiner, W.J. (1977b) Animal models of dyskinesia. In Hanin, I., Usdin, E. (eds.), *Animal Models in Psychiatry and Neurology.* New York: Pergamon Press, pp. 351–364.

Knapp, S., Mandell, A.J. (1976) Cocaine and lithium: Neurobiological antagonism in the serotonin biosynthetic system in rat brain. *Life Sci.* 18:679–683.

Kuczenski, R. (1983) Biochemical actions of amphetamine and other stimulants. In Creese, I. (ed.), *Stimulants: Neurochemical, Behavioral, and Clinical Perspectives.* New York: Raven Press, pp. 31–61.

Lesse, H. (1980) Prolonged effects of cocaine on hippocampal activity. *Commun. Psychopharmacol.* 4:247–254.

Lesse, H., Collins, J.P. (1980) Differential effects of cocaine on limbic excitability. *Pharmacol. Biochem. Behav.* 13:695–703.

McManus, C., Hartley, E.J., Seeman, P. (1978) Increased binding of

[³H]apomorphine in caudate membranes after dopamine pretreatment *in vitro. J. Pharm. Pharmacol.* 30:444–447.

Martin, W.R., Sloan, J.W., Sapira, J.D., Jasinski, D.R. (1971) Physiological subjective, and behavioral effects of amphetamine, methamphetamine, ephedrine, phenmetrazine, and methylphenidate in man. *Clin. Pharmacol. Ther.* 12:245–258.

Martres, M.P., Costenstin, J., Baudry, M., Marcais, H., Protais, P., Schwartz, J.C. (1977) Long-term changes in the sensitivity of pre- and postsynaptic dopamine receptors in mouse striatum evidenced by behavioural and biochemical studies. *Brain Res.* 136:319–337.

Matsuzaki, M., Spingler, P.J., Misra, A.L. (1976) Cocaine: tolerance to its convulsant and cardiorespiratory stimulating effects in the monkey. *Life Sci.* 19:193–203.

Memo, M., Pradhan, S., Hanbauer, I. (1981) Cocaine-induced supersensitivity of striatal dopamine receptors: role of endogenous calmodulin. *Neuropharmacol.* 20:1145–1150.

Misra, A.L. (1976) Disposition and biotransformation of cocaine. In Mule, S.J. (ed.), *Cocaine: Chemical, Biological, Clinical, Social and Treatment Aspects.* Cleveland: CRC Press, pp. 71–90.

Missale, C., Memo, M., Castelletti, L., Govoni, S., Trabucchi, M., Spano, P.F., Hanbauer, I. (1984) Different characteristics of ³H-cocaine binding sites in rat striatum and nucleus accumbens. *Society for Neuroscience Abstracts,* Vol. 10, 14th Annual Meeting, Anaheim, Calif., October 10–15, 1984, Abstr. No. 108.17, 1984.

Muller, P., Seeman, P. (1979) Presynaptic subsensitivity as a possible basis for sensitization by long-term dopamine mimetics. *Eur. J. Pharmacol.* 55:149–157.

Nielson, E.B., Nielsen, M., Ellison, G., Braestrup, C. (1980) Decreased spiroperidol and LSD binding on rat brain after continuous amphetamine. *Eur. J. Pharmacol.* 66:149–154.

Owen, F., Ridley, R., Baker, H., Crow, T.J. (1980) Chronic administration of amphetamine to monkeys: effects on receptors, neurotransmitters and related enzymes. *Abstracts of the 12th CINP Congress,* Goteborg, Sweden, June 22–26, 1980, Abstr. No. 509, pp. 274–275.

Pert, C.B., Pert, A., Rosenblatt, J.E., Tallman, J.F., Bunney, W.E. Jr. (1979) Catecholamine receptor stabilization: a possible mode of lithium's anti-manic action. In Usdin, E., Kopin, I.J., Barchas, J. (eds.), *Catecholamines: Basic and Clinical Frontiers.* New York: Pergamon Press, pp. 583–585.

Peterson, R. (1977) Cocaine: an overview. In Petersen, R., Stillman, R. (eds.), *Cocaine 1977.* NIDA Research Monograph N. 13. Washington, D.C.: U.S. Government Printing Office, pp. 5–16.

Peterson, S.L., Albertson, T.E. (1982) Neurotransmitter and neuro-modulator function in the kindled seiure and state. *Prog. Neurobiol.* 19:237–270.

Pettit, H.O., Ettenberg, A., Bloom, F.E., Koob, G.F. (1984) Destruction of dopamine in the nucleus accumbens selectively attenuates cocaine but not heroin self-administration in rats. *Psychopharmacol.* 84:167–173.

Pinel, J.P.J., Rovner, L.I. (1978a) Electrode placement and kindling-induced experimenta l epilepsy. *Exp. Neurol.* 58:335–346.

Pinel, J.P.J., Rovner, L.I. (1978b) Experimental epileptogenesis: Kindling-induced epilepsy in rats. *Exp. Neurol.* 58:190–202.

Post, R.M. (1981a) Lidocaine kindled limbic seizures: behavioral implications. In Wada, J.A. (ed.), *Kindling 2.* New York: Raven Press, pp. 149–160.

Post, R.M. (1981b) Central stimulants: clinical and experimental evidence on tolerance and sensitization. In Israel, Y., Galser, F.B., Kalant, H., Popham, R.E., Schmidt, W., Smart, R.G. (eds.), *Research Advances in Alcohol and Drug Problems,* Vol. 6. New York: Plenum, pp. 1–65.

Post, R.M. (1977) Progressive changes in behavior and seizures following chronic cocaine administration: relationship of kindling and psychosis. In Ellinwood, E.H., Kilbey, M.M. (eds.), *Advances in Behavioral Biology,* Vol. 21, *Cocaine and other Stimulants.* New York: Plenum, pp. 353–372.

Post, R.M. (1976) Clinical aspects of cocaine: assessment of acute and chronic effects in animals and man. In Mule, S.J. (ed.), *Cocaine: Chemical, Biological, Clinical, Social, and Treatment Aspects.* Cleveland: CRC Press, pp. 203–215.

Post, R.M. (1975) Cocaine psychoses: a continuum model. *Am. J. Psychiat.* 132:255–231.

Post, R.M., Ballenger, J.C. (1981) Kindling models for the progressive development of behavioral psychopathology: sensitization to electrical, pharmacological, and psychological stimuli. In van Praag, H.M., Lade, M.H., Rafaelsen, O.J., Sachar, E.J. (eds.), *Handbook of Biological Psychiatry,* part IV. New York: Marcel Dekker, pp. 609–651.

Post, R.M., Contel, N.R. (1983) Human and animal studies of cocaine: implications for development of behavioral pathology. In Creese, I. (ed.), *Stimulants: Neurochemical, Behavioral, and Clinical Perspective.* New York: Raven Press, pp. 169–203.

Post, R.M., Contel, N.R., Gold, P.W. (1982) Impaired behavioral sensitization to cocaine in vasopressin deficient rats. *Life Sci.* 31: 2745–2750.

Post, R.M., Kennedy, C., Shinohara, M. Squillace, K., Miyaoka, M.,

Suda, S., Ingvar, D.H., Sokoloff, L. (1979) Local cerebral glucose utilization in lidocaine-kindled seizures. In *Society for Neuroscience Abstracts*, Vol 5 (Abstr. No 646). Bethesda, Md.: Society for Neuroscience, p. 176.

Post, R.M., Kennedy, C., Shinohara, M., Squillace, K., Miyaoka, M., Suda, S., Ingvar, D.H., Sokoloff, L. (1984) Metabolic and behavioral consequences of lidocaine-kindled seizures. *Brain Res.* 324:295–304.

Post, R.M., Kopanda, R.T. (1976) Cocaine, kindling, and psychosis. *Am. J. Psychiat.* 133:627–634.

Post, R.M., Kopanda, R.T., Black, K.E. (1976) Progressive effects of cocaine on behavior and central amine metabolism in rhesus monkeys: relationship to kindling and psychoses. *Biol Psychiat.* 11:403–419.

Post, R.M., Kopanda, R.T., Lee, A. (1975) Progressive behavioral changes during chronic lidocaine administration: relationship to kindling. *Life Sci* 17:943–950.

Post, R.M., Kotin, J., Goodwin, F.K. (1974) The effects of cocaine on depressed patients. *Am. J. Psychiat.* 131:511–517.

Post, R.M., Lockfeld, A., Squillace, K.M., Contel N.R. (1981a) Drug-evironment interaction: context dependency of cocaine-induced behavioral sensitization. *Life Sci.* 28:755–760.

Post, R.M., Rubinow, D.R., Ballenger, J.C. (1984a) Conditioning, sensitization, and kindling: implications for the course of affective illness. In Post, R.M., Ballenger, J.C. (eds.) *Neurobiology of Mood Disorders.* Baltimore: Williams & Wilkins, pp. 432–466.

Post, R.M., Squillace, K.M., Pert, A., Sass, W. (1981b) Effect of amygdala kindling on spontaneous and cocaine-induced motor activity and lidocaine seizures. *Psychopharmacol.* 72:189–196.

Post, R.M., Squillace, K.M., Sass, W., Pert, A. (1977) Drug sensitization and electrical kindling. In *Society for Neuroscience Abstracts*, Vol. 3 (Abstr. No. 637). Bethesda, Md.: Society for Neuroscience, p. 204.

Post, R.M., Weiss, S.R.B., Pert, A. (1984b) Differential effects of carbamazepine and lithium on sensitization and kindling. *Prog. Neuropsychopharmacol. Biol. Psychiat.* 8:425–434.

Pycock, C., Dawborn, D., O'Shaughnesy, C. (1982) Behavioural and biochemical changes following chronic administration of L-dopa to rats. *Eur. J. Pharmacol.* 79:201–215.

Quik, M., Iversen, I. (1978) Subsensitivity of the rat striatal dopaminergic system after treatment with bromocriptine: effects on ^{3}H-spiperone binding and dopamine-stimulated cyclic AMP formation. *Naunyn-Schmiedebergs Arch. Pharmacol.* 301:141–145.

Racine, R. (1978) Kindling: the first decade. *Neurosurgery* 3:234–252.

Racine, R., Livingston, K., Joaquin, A. (1975) Effects of procaine hydrochloride, diazepam, and diphenylhydantoin on seizure development in cortical and subcortical structures in rats. *Electroencephalogr. Clin. Neurophysiol.* 38:355–365.

Rebec, G.V., Segal, D.S. (1980) Apparent tolerance to some aspects of amphetamine stereotypy with long-term treatment. *Pharmacol. Biochem. Behav.* 13:792–797.

Reith, M.E.A., Allen, D.L., Sershen, H., Lajtha, A. (1984) Similarities and differences between high-affinity binding sites for cocaine and imipramine in mouse cerebral cortex. *J. Neurochem.* 43:249–255.

Reith, M.E.A., Sershen, H., Allen, D.L., Lajtha, A. (1983) A portion of [^{3}H] cocaine binding in brain is associated with serotonergic neurons. *Mol. Pharmacol.* 23:600–606.

Reith, M.E.A., Sershen, H., Lajtha, A. (1981) Binding of [^{3}H] cocaine in mouse brain: kinetics and saturability. *J. Recept. Res.* 2:233–243.

Resnick, R.B., Kestenbaum, R.S., Schwartz, L.K. (1977) Acute systemic effects of cocaine in man: a controlled study of intranasal and intravenous routes. *Science* 195:696–698.

Ridley, R.M., Baker, H.F., Owen, F., Cross, A.J., Crow, T.J. (1982) Behavioural and biochemical effects of chronic amphetamine treatment in the vervet monkey. *Psychopharmacol.* 78:245–251.

Riffee, W.H., Wilcox, R.E., Vaughn, D.M., Smith, R.V. (1982) Dopamine receptor sensitivity after chronic dopamine agonists striatal ^{3}H-spiroperidol binding in mice after chronic administration of high doses of apomorphine, n-n-propylnorapomorphine and dextroamphetamine. *Psychopharmacol.* 77:146–149.

Roberts, D.C.S., Koob, G.F., Klonoff, P., Fibiger, H.C. (1980) Extinction and recovery of cocaine self-administration following 6-hydroxydopamine lesions of the nucleus accumbens. *Pharmacol. Biochem. Behav.* 12:781–787.

Robertson, H.A. (1980) Stimulation of ^{3}H-apomorphine binding by dopamine and bromocriptine. *Eur. J. Pharmacol.* 61:209–211.

Robertson, H.A. (1979) Effect of chronic d-amphetamine or beta-phenylethylamine on dopamine binding in rat striatum and limbic system. *Proceeding's 9th Annual Meeting*, Society for Neuroscience, Atlanta, Abstr. No. 1936, p. 570.

Robinson, T.E., Becker, J.B. (1982) Behavioral sensitization is accompanied by an enhancement in amphetamine-stimulated dopamine release from striatal tissue *in vitro. Eur. J. Pharmacol.* 85:253–254.

Ross, S.B., Renyi, A.L. (1966) Uptake of some tritiated sympathomimetic amines by mouse brain cortex slices *in vitro. Acta. Pharmacol. Toxicol.* 24: 297–309.

Sahakian, B.J., Carlson, K.R., DeGirolami, U., Bhawan, J. (1980) Functional and structural consequences of long-term dietary 1-dopa treatment in mice. *Commun. Psychopharmacol.* 4:169–176.

Sato, M., Tomoda, T., Hikasa, N., Otsuki, S. (1980) Inhibition of amygdaloid kindling by chronic pretreatment with cocaine or methamphetamine. *Epilepsia* 21:497–507.

Scheel-Kruger, J., Braestrup, C., Nielson, M., Golembrowska, K., Mogilnicka, E. (1977) Cocaine: discussion on the role of dopamine in the biochemical mechanism of action. In Ellinwood, E.H., Kilbey, M.M. (eds.) *Advances in Behavioral Biology*, Vol. 21, *Cocaine and Other Stiomulants*. New York: Plenum Press, pp. 373–408.

Schiff, S.R., Bridger, W.H. (1978) Conditioned dopaminergic activity—behavioral, pharmacological and biochemical evidence. 11th Congress CINP, Vienna, July 9–14, 1978, p. 114.

Schwartz, J.C., Castentin, J., Martres, M.P., Protais, P., Baudry, M. (1978) Modulation of receptor mechanisms in the CNS: hyper- and hyposensitivity to catecholamines. *Neuropharmacol.* 17:665–685.

Segal, D.S., Schuckit, M.A. (1983) Animal models of stimulent-induced psychosis. In Creese, I. (ed.) *Stimulants: Neurochemical, Behavioral, and Clinical Perspectives*. New York: Raven Press, pp. 131–167.

Sershen, H., Reith, M.E.A., Lajtha, A. (1982) Comparison of the properties of central and peripheral binding sites for cocaine. *Neuropharmacol.* 21:469–474.

Sershen, H., Reith, M.E.A., Lajtha, A. (1980) The pharmacological relevance of the cocaine binding site in mouse brain. *Neuropharmacol.* 19: 1145–1148.

Shearman, G.T., Lal, H. (1981) Discriminative stimulus properties of cocaine related to an anxiogenic action. *Prog. Neuropsychopharmacol.* 5:57–63.

Shuster, L., Yu, G., Bates, A. (1977) Sensitization to cocaine stimulation in mice. *Psychopharmacol.* 52:185–190.

Siegel, R.K. (1977) Cocaine: recreational use and intoxication. In Petersen, R.C., Stillman, R.C. (eds.), Cocaine: 1977. NIDA Research Monograph No. 13. Washington, D.C.: U.S. Government Printing Office, pp. 119–136.

Siegel, R.K. (1984) Changing patterns of cocaine use: longitudinal observations, consequences, and treatment. In Grabowski, J. (ed.), *Cocaine: Pharmacology, Effects and Treatment of Abuse*. NIDA Research Monograph No. 50. Washington, D.C.: U.S. Government Printing Office, pp. 92–110.

Squillace, K.M., Post, R.M., Pert, A. (1982) Effect of lidocaine pretreatment on cocaine-induced behavior in normal and amygdala-lesioned rats. *Neuropsychol.* 8:113–122.

Stripling, J.S., Hendricks, C. (1982) Effect of cocaine on afterdischarge threshold in previously kindled rats. *Pharmacol. Biochem. Behav.* 16:855–857.

Szostak, C., Martin-Iversen, M.T., Fibiger, H.C. (1984) Effects of 6-hydroxydopamine lesions of the medial prefrontal cortex on cocaine self-administration. *Society for Neuroscience Abstracts*, Vo. 10, 14th Annual Meeting, Anaheim, Calif., October 10–15, 1984, Abstr. No. 337.7, p. 1167.

Tatum, A.L., Seevers, M.H. (1929) Experimental cocaine addiction. *J. Pharmacol. Exp. Ther.* 36;401–410.

Taylor, D.L., Ho, B.T., Fagan, J.D. (1979) Increased dopamine receptor binding in rat brain by repeated cocaine injections. *Commun. Psychopharmacol.* 3:137–142.

Thiebot, M.-H., Kloczko, J., Chermat, R., Peuch, A.J., Soubrie, P., Simon, P. (1981) Enhancement of cocaine-induced hyperactivity in mice by benzodiazepines: evidence for an interaction of GABAergic processes with catecholaminergic neurons? *Eur. J. Pharmacol.* 76: 335–343.

Toth-Kennedy, L., Hanbauer, I. (1983) Sodium-sensitive cocaine binding to rat striatal membrane: possible relationship to dopamine uptake sites. *J. Neurochem.* 41:172–178.

Trulson, M.E., Jacobs, B.L. (1979) Long-term amphetamine treatment decreases brain serotonin metabolism: implications for theories of schizophrenia. *Science* 205:1295–1297.

Uhde, T.W., Boulenger, J.P., Roy-Byrne, P.P., Vittone, B.J., Post, R.M. (1985) Longitudinal couse of panic disorder: clinical and biological considerations. *Prog. Neuropsychopharmacol. Biol. Psychiat.* 9:39–51.

Van Dyke, C., Jatlow, P., Ungerer, J., Barash, P., Byck, R. (1979) Cocaine and lidocaine have similar psychological effects after intranasal application. *Life Sci.* 24:271–274.

van Rossum, J.M. (1970) Mode of action of psychomotor stimulants. *Int. Rev. Neurobiol.* 12:307–383.

Wada, J.A., Sato, M. (1974) Generalized convulsive seizures induced by daily electrical stimulation of the amygdala in cats. *Neurology* 24:565–574.

Wada, J.A., Sato, M., Corcoran, M.E. (1974) Persistent seizure susceptibility and recurrent spontaneous seizures in kindled cats. *Epilepsia* 15:465–478.

Wagman, I.H., de Jong, R.H., Prince, D.A. (1967) Effects of lidocaine on the central nervous system. *Anesthesiology* 28:155–172.

Washton, A.M., Gold, M.S. (1984) Chronic cocaine abuse: evidence for adverse effects on health and functioning. *Psychiatr. Ann.* 14:733–743.

Washton, A.M., Tatarsky, A. (1984) Adverse effects of cocaine abuse. In Harris, L.S. (ed.), *Problems of Drug Dependence, 1983.* NIDA Research Monograph No. 49. Washington, D.C.: U.S. Government Printing Office, pp. 247–254.

Wesson, D.R., Smith, D.F. (1977) Cocaine: its use for central nervous system stimulation including recreational and medical uses. In Petersen, R.C., Stillman, R.C. (eds.) *Cocaine: 1977.* NIDA Research Monograph No. 13. Washington, D.C.: U.S. Government Printing Office, pp. 137–152.

White, F.J., Wang, R.Y. (1984) Electrophysiological evidence for A10 dopamine autoreceptor subsensitivity following chronic d-amphetamine treatment. *Brain Res.* 309:283–292.

Wilner, K.D., Butler, I.J., Seifert, W.E., Clement-Cormier, Y.C. (1980) Biochemical alterations of dopamine receptor responses following chronic L-dopa therapy. *Biochem. Pharmacol.* 29:701–706.

Wirz-Justice, A. (1983) Amphetamine and circadian rhythms. CPB-NIMH Lecture. Bethesda, Md., June 9, 1983.

Wise, R.A. (1984) Neural mechanisms of the reinforcing action of cocaine. In Grabowski, J. (ed.), *Cocaine: Pharmacology, Effects, and Treatment of Abuse.* NIDA Monograph Series No. 50. Washington, D.C.: U.S. Government Printing Office, pp. 15–33.

Woolverton, W.L., Balster, R.L. (1979) Reinforcing properties of some local anesthetics in rhesus monkeys. *Pharmacol. Biochem. Behav.* 11:669–672.

Woolverton, W.L., Kandel, D., Schuster, C.R. (1978) Tolerance and cross-tolerance to cocaine and d-amphetamine. *J. Pharmacol. Exp. Ther.* 205:525–535.

6 | Issues in Cocaine-Abuse Treatment Research

FRANK H. GAWIN and HERBERT KLEBER

SCIENTIFIC evaluation of cocaine abuse and its treatment is sparse. No consensus exists on optimal treatment strategies. We summarize here current treatments and preliminary data on new approaches, as well as frame issues that will require attention before rigorous scientific comparisons of treatment modalities can be achieved.

The clinical data reviewed here is based only on patients who receive treatment. Cocaine abuse, like any other excess, can sometimes be controlled without treatment, but such experiences have not been systematically examined. Also, investigations of cocaine-abuse treatment are just getting underway, so only clinical observations and preliminary systematic research are available for this review.

COCAINE ABUSERS

DSM-III does not list cocaine dependence since, when written, it was believed that the two cardinal manifestations of "classic" drug dependence—either tolerance or withdrawal—were not brought about by chronic cocaine use. DSM-III does list amphetamine dependence. As the quantity and quality of cocaine used has increased, clinicians now describe what appears to be tolerance and withdrawal in heavy users, especially among freebase smokers or intravenous users, similar to that observed with amphetamine. However, recent clinical observations indicate that "classic" drug dependence categorizations may not be clinically useful for modern cocaine abusers (Gawin & Kleber, 1985b).

Individuals who abuse cocaine do not form a homogeneous class. Distinctions on two dimensions of abuse have clear treatment relevance: intensity of cocaine use and psychiatric symptomatology.

Intensity of Use

There may be greater variation in severity of use for cocaine abusers than in patients seeking treatment for abuse of other substances (Kleber & Gawin, 1984; Gold, 1983). Like marijuana, cocaine had been labelled by popular culture as "recreational." Until recently, most who tried cocaine did so believing that they would have no difficulty controlling their use. Many people apparently do maintain control. Some, however, do not and appear for treatment. The point at which treatment is sought varies greatly. Because of cocaine's expense, significant psychosocial disruption leading to treatment can occur without significant dependence (Byck, this volume). At the other end of the cocaine abuse spectrum lie very heavy intravenous or free-base cocaine abusers (Siegel, 1982), who use cocaine continuously for prolonged periods in a pattern very similar to i.v. metamphetamine addicts observed over a decade ago (Kramer, 1967). Several studies have established that severe cocaine abuse can develop with any route of administration (Gawin & Kleber, 1985a; Helfrich et al., 1983; Weiss et al., 1983), although clinical consensus is that intravenous abusers or cocaine free-base smokers are more likely to develop significant distress requiring treatment. There are no epidemiologic studies comparing distress and need for treatment with mode of administration, so this assertion has not been tested. Because route of administration is an incomplete indicator of severity, other factors, such as amount of use, pattern and duration of use, degree of psychosocial disruption and impairment of impulse control, medical and psychiatric characteristics, as well as prior treatment attempts and treatment response all also require consideration. Treatment needs vary based on the severity of dependence and the status of all these factors. Careful clinical judgments and flexibility are therefore necessary in cocaine abuse treatment programs.

Psychiatric Symptomatology

Accurate psychiatric characterization of the cocaine abuser is important because symptomatology preceding abuse or appearing during abstinence can indicate the need for trials of pharmacological adjuncts.

Only two studies using DSM-III criteria and structured diagnostic interviews have been reported. Weiss et al. (1983) presented data on 30 hospitalized cocaine abusers and the authors (Gawin & Kleber, 1985b) reported Axis I data on 30 outpatient cocaine abusers. These independent studies generated very similar results: depressive disorders (Major Depression, Dysthymic Disorder, Atypical Depression) appeared in 30 percent and bipolar disorders (especially Cyclothymic Disorder) in approximately 20% of each sample. Also, a smaller (less than 10%) but possibly important subgroup of patients with ADD-residual type were found in each sample. Thus, a significant proportion of cocaine abusers could be self-medicating. If so, conventional pharmacotherapies could replace cocaine as self-medication of Axis I symptoms.

This conclusion, however, may be partially misleading. First, symptoms may be a consequence of abuse, not the cause, and may not respond to medications effective in similar primary psychiatric disorders. Second, differentiating between the acute, short-lived depressive symptomatology following each binge of cocaine use (the post-cocaine "crash") and enduring symptoms that are independent of individual episodes of cocaine use is difficult. Diagnostic studies have attempted to circumvent these issues by gathering extensive historical data and family history data, and by requiring that symptom assessments occur only during abstinence periods that are isolated from acute cocaine use and acute post-cocaine depression. In the absence of prospective studies etiological questions cannot be answered, but diagnostic categories may nonetheless tentatively guide treatment. The medication responsiveness of symptoms observed in abusers with Axis 1 diagnoses in a subject of ongoing investigation in our clinic and is discussed further below. It should be noted that our diagnostic data and those of Weiss et al. (1983) differ markedly from Smith's (1984) and others' estimates, which are not based on systematic assessments or structured interviews, that 90% of cocaine abusers do not have Axis I diagnoses. This may illustrate a bias introduced by treatment site (e.g., psychiatric facility vs. walk-in clinic), and points out the necessity for structured diagnostic assessments to compare samples across treatment settings.

CURRENT TREATMENTS

Because cocaine dependence has long been considered "psychological," current treatments usually consist of psychological strategies aimed at modifying addictive behaviors. Almost all psychotherapeutic treatment of cocaine abusers can be organized around three dimensions: behavioral, supportive, and psychodynamic (Kleber & Gawin, 1984).

Behavioral

This dimension utilizes the abuser's ability to respond to deleterious effects of cocaine use and accept the need to stop that use. Occasional cocaine users usually do not seek treatment. The vast majority of those seeking help find cocaine use has become a central part of their life. They are usually ambivalent. Many have an inner conviction that cocaine harms them, but they still hope they can control their drug use and do not want to give up drug-induced euphoria. Often marked external pressure from family members, employers, or legal pressures forces them to come for treatment. If these clients are to remain in treatment, psychotherapy must address this ambivalence early on.

Anker and Crowley (1982) have adapted the behavioral method of contingency contracting for cocaine abuse. This method focuses and magnifies cocaine's aversive effects. The approach has two basic elements: agreement to participate in a urine-monitoring program; and attachment of an aversive contingency to either a cocaine-positive urine or a failure to produce a scheduled urine sample. The aversive contingencies are derived from the patient's own statements of the adverse consequences expected to result from continued cocaine use. This adverse effect is then scheduled to occur at the very next use of cocaine. For example, a letter with irrevocable personal consequences, admitting to cocaine abuse and addressed to the patient's employer or professional licensing board, is held by the therapist and is mailed in the event of positive urinalysis or missed urinalysis. Such contracts, coupled with supportive psychotherapy, appear to be effective as long as patients are willing to take part. Anker and Crowley report 48% of their sample (32 of 67 pts) were willing to engage in this treatment, with over 80% cocaine abstinence during the duration of the "contract" which averaged 3 months. However, over half of these patients relapsed following completion of the contract (Crowley, 1982). Patients refusing to enter into contracts (52%) were treated with supportive psychotherapy alone, but over 90% of these patients dropped out and/or resumed cocaine abuse within two to four weeks. Anker and Crowley presented no comparisons of severity of cocaine use between patients who were willing or unwilling to use "contracts," and thus ignore the likely possibility that cocaine abusers with severe craving and problems of control recognize their inability to comply and consequently avoid contingency treatment. In addition to limited long-term efficacy and possible inapplicability to more severe cocaine abuse, there are potential ethical problems existing in those cases where less damaging procedures could have been attempted.

The major lesson from the contingency contracting approach is straightforward: it focuses and magnifies the actual self-harm from cocaine abuse. The clear emphasis this method gives to the deleterious effects of cocaine abuse can be replicated in conventional individual, group, and family psychotherapy in a less potentially harmful manner than contingency contracts. Less severe contingencies could be employed in a gradual escalation, as could positive contingencies—for example, starting with a sum of money from the patient and releasing part each week for clean urines. Some cases might optimally need a combination of both positive and negative reinforcement. Research into reinforcement design is clearly needed. None of these variations on contingency contracting has been systematically evaluated in stimulant abusers.

Supportive

This approach emphasizes disassociating the abuser from cocaine use situations and cocaine sources in initial limit setting, and helping the abuser ultimately manage impulsive behavior in general and cocaine use in particular. Siegel (1982) describes using frequent supportive psychotherapy sessions, self-control strategies, "exercise therapy," and liberal use of hospitalization during initial "detoxification." This treatment first separates the user from the use-fostering environment via external controls, and then gradually facilitates internalization of controls through psychotherapy. Half of Siegel's sample of 32 heavy cocaine smokers dropped out, but 80% of those remaining were cocaine-free at nine month follow-up. Recently, Washton et al. (1985) have reported success with a similar approach in a larger outpatient sample.

Anker and Crowley (1982) also employ supportive approaches, considering key points to be: encouraging increased contact with nonusing friends; eliminating paraphernalia and drug stashes; terminating relationships with dealers; changing phone numbers, or even residence if needed, to stop drug-related calls and visits; counseling with spouses; and examining relating problem areas in the patient's life.

Whether only cocaine is to be stopped, or all mood-altering substances, is controversial. When a patient has not had a problem with alcohol or marijuana in the past, they usually want to continue such use. Clinical cases indicate cocaine abstinence can occur in the context of a pre-cocaine level of recreational substance use for some abusers. But Alcoholics Anonymous, Narcotics Anonymous, or Cocaine Anonymous related programs usually insist on the total cessation of all mood-altering drugs, excluding nicotine and caffeine, on the reasonable basis that the patient has demonstrated addictive tendencies. Another important reason for a total abstinence model is that patients often find craving increases in the context of conditioned cues for cocaine, and that one of the most powerful of such cues is other intoxicants which were previously paired with cocaine; particularly alcohol. It is not clear how to predict who requires a total abstinence approach. Patients who require total abstinence often learn this lesson firsthand by relapsing before they become willing to give up other drugs.

Self-help groups based on a total abstinence approach such as N.A., and more recently C.A., also provide structure, limits, and a helping network. They thus employ both supportive and behavioral techniques. Although they have been described as effective, they have not been the subject of outcome studies in cocaine abuse.

Psychodynamic

Psychodynamic treatment approaches aim toward understanding the functions that cocaine has played in the abuser's life and to help him or her serve these functions without drugs (Wurmser, 1974). Cocaine use serves a variety of needs: narcissistic needs are often served by the glamour associated with cocaine use; the cocaine-using subculture may provide a sense of identity; anaclitic needs can be met via cocaine-heightened intimacy; cocaine may be used to compensate for interpersonal failures; the use and obtaining of cocaine may substitute for inadequate leisure alternatives; cocaine may be used to cope with a sense of inner emptiness and existential issues; and, finally, cocaine serves to manage multiple other symptoms. The understanding of cocaine's relationship to specific needs may lead to more constructive substitutes. Understanding also provides an increased sense of control in the abuser, which then limits the need to turn to cocaine euphoria for an illusory sense of power and control, and also provides self-monitoring tools that help the abuser predict and deter potential relapse.

A combination of all three orientations—behavioral, supportive, and psychodynamic—is probably the most common form of treatment for both inpatient and outpatient settings. The optimal admixture of these orientations is best determined by considering the needs of the individual cocaine abuser at the time of seeking treatment, rather than by preexisting program structure (which most often defines treatment design in current treatment settings). For example, severe cocaine abusers attempting abstinence are often too dysphoric to respond to psychodynamic interventions, while moderate abusers seem more readily able to utilize them. Also, the mild abuser may need little more than clarification of the consequences of abuse, using mild contingency methods, to stop cocaine use. Hence, choice of primary therapeutic orientation might shift from behavioral to psychodynamic to supportive as severity increases. Neither these notions of matching the treatment to severity or the value of using any specific supportive or psychodynamic techniques have as yet received any systematic empirical testing.

Whether inpatient or outpatient treatment is indicated, and for whom, is also unresolved and requires further study. Siegel (1982) as well as others (AMA Council on Scientific Affairs, 1978; Connell, 1970) strongly favor hospitalization for initial stimulant abuse detoxification. However, in our recent studies using pharmacologic agents (Kleber & Gawin, 1984), as well as in nonpharmacological studies by Anker and Crowley (1982), little need for hospitalization was evident. This may reflect differences in treatment variables. For example, Siegel treated heavy cocaine smokers with minimal pharmacotherapy, and pharmacotherapy may have controlled symptoms in our studies that would otherwise have required hospitalization. The only clearly accepted factors indicating need for inpatient cocaine abuse treatment are severe depression or psychotic symptoms lasting beyond the one to three days of the post-cocaine "crash," or repeated outpatient treatment failures. Other factors remain controversial. Washton et al. (1985) have summarized the reasons for hospitalization as follows:

1. Concurrent dependence on alcohol or other drugs (in this case, the hospitalization is primarily for withdrawal of the other substance).
2. Psychiatric or medical problems of a serious nature.
3. Repeated outpatient failures.
4. Chronic free base or i.v. use, "because the use is, usually, out of control."
5. Psychosocial impairment of a severe nature.
6. Lack of motivation.
7. Lack of family or social supports.

We agree with Washton et al. on points one to three, but feel the last four criteria may be used too often for unnecessary hospitalization. Our clinical impressions, gained on work with severe abusers, lead us to favor outpatient treatment. Since the cocaine abuser must resume everyday life at some point, hospitalization merely defers this point. Both studies of animal behavior (Goldberg et al., 1979; Spellman et al., 1977), and clinical work with humans (Maddux & Desmond, 1982; Wikler, 1973), highlight the importance of environment in conditioning drug-taking behavior. Cocaine craving can also become strongly conditioned to otherwise innocuous environmental stimuli temporally associated with past cocaine use. Such conditioned cues, as varied as geographic locations, interpersonal strife, periods free from work or family, objects with potential to be paraphenalia, and many others, must be an active focus of treatment efforts at extinction. We have observed that a period of abstinence akin to a period of "extinction," within the context of everyday stimuli, cues, stressors, and consequent craving, is necessary before long-term reduction in cocaine craving occurs. The current almost ubiquitous presence of cocaine in many areas of American life makes it unlikely that the former user will be abel to simply avoid temptation. Like the former cigarette smoker or alcoholic, the person attempting to give up cocaine must make the drug "psychologically" unavailable since it is so hard in current society to ensure that it be permanently physically unavailable.

EXPERIMENTAL PHARMACOLOGICAL TREATMENTS

Findings from neurotransmitter, neuroreceptor, and electrophysiological studies of chronic cocaine and similar stimulants in animals suggest that neuroadaptation may occur in cocaine abuse, and that various pharmacologic agents might be useful in treatment. In the forefront of current investigations are tricyclic antidepressants, lithium carbonate, and methylphenidate.

These agents could each facilitate cocaine abstinence by two different mechanisms. The following discussion pertains to the possible use of these agents first as general treatments, irrespective of distinctions in symptomatology, and then as specific treatments for particular subpopulations of cocaine abusers.

Tricyclic Antidepressants (TCAs)

Animal research on chronic cocaine administration suggests long-term neurophysiological changes occur that may be reversible by treatment with TCAs. Several reports indicate that treatment with TCA's reverses the decrease in animal self-stimulation reward indices (Simpson, 1974; Kokkinidis et al., 1980; Fibiger et al., 1981) that follows chronic stimulant administration. This presents a possible animal model for human stimulant craving and anhedonia as well as their treatment. Studies of receptor changes in animals report increased beta-adrenergic (Banerjee et al., 1979; Chanda et al., 1979; Pert et al., 1979) and dopaminergic (Borison et al., 1979; Taylor et al., 1979) receptor binding. Receptor supersensitivity (beta-adrenergic or dopaminergic) could be a neurochemical substrate for post-cocaine dysphoria or craving. In a preliminary study, the authors reported some human cocaine abusers have elevated plasma growth hormone and decreased plasma prolactin (Gawin & Kleber, 1985c), findings that may be consistent with the receptor changes in animals. Beta-adrenergic supersensitivity has been hypothesized to be a cause of depressive illness and beta-adrenergic subsensitivity follows antidepressant treatments, possibly explaining their mechanism of action (Charney et al., 1981; Maggi et al.,

1980). Dopaminergic receptor changes following antidepressant treatment (Koide et al., 1981; Naber et al., 1980) also are in the opposite direction of those occuring following chronic cocaine use, and could be even more important since dopamine may mediate acute cocaine euphoria (Wise, 1980) and the craving, dysphoria, or anhedonia seen after chronic cocaine could be based on adaptations within dopaminergic systems.

These studies lend neurochemical plausibility to the clinical observation that TCA therapy can be helpful in treating the depressed stimulant abuser (Ellinwood, 1977). We have recently reported prolonged (>12 weeks) abstinence with desipramine treatment in eleven of twelve subjects (Gawin & Kleber, 1984). Craving decreases followed a time course consistent with desipramine's time course for neuroreceptor changes and its known clinical characteristics in depressive disorders. Most of the subjects *did not* meet criteria for major depressive disorder and displayed desipramine-associated craving decreases and abstinence-facilitating effects despite the absence of significant depression. All were prior nonpharmacological treatment failures.

Prior to our study, Tennant and Rawson (1983) reported anecdotal data that desipramine briefly facilitated treatment in 14 cocaine abusers. Their study was based on the rationale involving acute desipramine-induced decreases in catecholamine reuptake rather than receptor changes; consequently, 11 of their 14 subjects received desipramine less than 7 days. A subsequent case report indicated desipramine might alleviate symptoms of the post-cocaine crash (Baxter, 1983). This has not been reported by our subjects, and neither of these short-term treatment effects was confirmed in a later double-blind study by Tenant and Rawson (1985).

Rosecan (1985a) has also reported an open clinical trial using imipramine, L-tyrosine and L-tryptophan with cocaine abusers. Twenty of twenty-five patients either markedly decreased or stopped using cocaine completely over 10 weeks. In preliminary investigations, he has also reported a diminution of the cocaine high which appeared to be dose related (Rosecan, 1985b). We have not observed consistent effects on the cocaine high using desipramine.

Although the above results on long-term TCA's as a general cocaine-abuse treatment are encouraging, the clinical reports cited are nonblind and uncontrolled. Controlled double-blind studies with larger samples are needed before any conclusions are drawn regarding desipramine or other trycyclics as a general treatment in cocaine abuse treatment.

Lithium Carbonate

Lithium carbonate treatment has been advocated for stimulant abuse based on lithium's antagonism of multiple acute stimulant effects including euphoria. Lithium blocks behavioral, electrophysiological, and neurochemical effects of acute cocaine and amphetamine in animals (Kleber et al., 1984). In several case studies (Cronson & Flemenbaum, 1978; Mandell & Knapp, 1976) lithium attenuated cocaine-induced euphoria, but lithium did not block IV cocaine euphoria in an experiment done on six methadone-treated opiate addicts with significant cocaine abuse (Resnick et al., 1977). In the latter study (not a direct treatment evaluation), lithium administration was associated with anecdotal reports of decreases in cocaine abuse, despite the lack of euphoria-attenuating effects.

In a report by the authors (Gawin & Kleber, 1984), three cyclothymic subjects treated with lithium stopped cocaine use while three noncyclothymic patients similarly treated did not. The non-responding patients reported cocaine euphoria was unchanged in intensity after lithium. Prior investigators have not considered that lithium might be useful in some cocaine abusers via a mechanism other than blockade of euphoria. Lithium may modulate fluctuations in functional receptor activity (Bunney et al., 1983). Lithium's effectiveness in bipolar patients could be due to damping of abnormal oscillations of select neuroreceptor populations (Bunney et al., 1977). Lithium might thus reverse cocaine-induced neurophysiologic changes. Further, if cocaine abuse causes receptor changes, bipolar or cyclothymic patients might be more sensitive to both such cocaine effects and to opposite lithium effects, possibly explaining the diagnostic specificity observed. In all, it is too early to draw any conclusions regarding lithium's efficacy, diagnostic specificity, or possible mechanisms of action in cocaine-abuse treatment. All require further study.

Methylphenidate (MPH)

Since methylphenidate produces euphoria indistinguishable from amphetamine (Brown et al., 1978) and, presumably, cocaine, in humans as well as cross-tolerance in animals, the authors thought MPH might produce clinically useful acute tolerance to other stimulants. Through such an acute "cross-tolerance," a given dose of cocaine would be less euphorigenic and have less abuse liability. This is similar to high dose methadone maintenance causing longer term tolerance to opiates, thereby reducing heroin euphoria and abuse. Unlike methadone, however, MPH tolerance would end sooner, requiring more frequent readministration due to its shorter half-life. Although MPH is an abusable euphorigen, it has the advantages of medical dispensation which include controlled dosage, decreased legal risk, economic stabilization and a breaking of "street" associations and secondary abuse reinforcers. In a pilot study done on 5 subjects, cocaine abusers considered it far less desirable than cocaine, and deteriorated during methlphenidate treatment; none became abstinent.

Six cocaine abusers with diagnoses of Attention Deficit Disorder (ADD), Residual Type, have been reported as successfully treated (Weiss et al., 1983; Khantzian, 1983) with either methylphenidate (4 cases) or pemoline (2 cases). In trial cases with an ADD diagnosis, the authors have had similar experience. Methylphenidate apparently has little practical potential as a general treatment for cocaine abusers, but its use in the context of ADD requires serious consideration and further investigation.

The potential pharmacotherapies described above simply represent the optimal treatment rationales available given the state of current theory and research. Much is unknown, and many other possibilities exist, including: peptides that putatively modulate dopaminergic transmission such as Arginine Vasopression analogues (Fraenkel et al., 1983), and CCK analogues and antagonists; coenzymes in dopaminergic synthesis such as pridoxine; or dopamine degradation inhibitors such as the MAO-B inhibitor deprenyl; neurotransmitter procursors such as tyrosine or tryptophan (Rosecan, 1985a; Gold et al., 1983); other indirect or direct dopamine agonists, and atypical antidepressants with substantial dopaminergic effects (such as nomifensine or bupropion) among numerous others.

ISSUES IN RESEARCH

It is difficult to contrast and assess the summarized studies of pharmacological and psychotherapeutic cocaine-abuse treatment, not only because they are preliminary efforts, but also because cocaine-abuse treatment research is particularly vulnerable to obscuring consequences of differences in study design. We summarize here methodological points that will require clarification and consensus before more definitive future studies can create a coherant body of scientifically acceptable research for cocaine-abuse treatment.

Severity

As noted, it is now clear that route of administration does not provide a simple barometer of abuse severity (Kleber et al., 1984). No treatment studies reported thus far have stratified samples according to any criteria of abuse severity. At least one study (Gawin & Kleber, 1984) has attempted to acknowledge differences in severity by evaluating a sample including only prior treatment failures, but that study did not contrast this to a sample without such a history. Most studies have provided data allowing comparisons of sociodemographic, psychometric (MMPI), or symptom variables between studies, but whether this data provides any meaningful distinctions for treatment design has not been determined. Further, no consensus on how to judge impairment or refractoriness to treatment has emerged. The psychotherapy treatment studies described thus far (Siegel, 1982; Anker et al., 1982, Washton, this volume) have a substantial proportion of early drop-outs or patients eliminated at screening who have not been contrasted to those remaining in treatment. Data describing not only the population in treatment and those responding to treatment, but also the populations that find particular treatments aversive or inadequate are obviously needed. No biological criteria for severity have emerged. One study (Gawin & Kleber, 1985a) indicates that as cocaine usage escalates, patterns of abuse change from controlled daily intake to uncontrolled use in binges extending several days, and abuse patterns may ultimately provide a useful index of severity. At present, however, severity remains difficult to operationalize, and present attempts to contrast sample populations may best rely on the generation of detailed and broad data on sample characteristics, in the hope that clear indicators of abuse severity will eventually emerge to retrospectively allow meaningful comparisons across studies.

Recovery

There is no consensus regarding how long abstinence must endure before recovery occurs or when treatment can end. Similarly, controversy not only exists regarding whether continued use of nonstimulant substances constitutes treatment failure, but also regarding whether, how much, and in whom such use increases risk of relapse. Further, no data exists on whether reduction but not elimination of cocaine use is a rational goal, or on whether only temporary breaks in use, brought about by hospitalization or periods in active treatment, contributes favorably to long-term outcome. In addition, no studies as yet have reported outcome in terms of changes in indices of psychosocial functioning, rather than by simply cataloguing decreased cocaine use. Not only are long-term follow-up studies crucial, but clear, comparable, and sufficiently broad definitions of outcome criteria are essential.

Heterogeneity

Multiple sources of sample heterogeneity exist that require attention in cocaine treatment populations. Variations in patterns and duration of use, severity of impairment, treatment history, and in other substances of abuse, and other factors may define subpopulations with potentially different treatment needs. One parameter already noted in pharmacological treatment trials is psychiatric diagnosis. Some programs stratify treatment groups according to socioeconomic or professional status. Whether this is beneficial has not been empirically studied.

Etiology, Course, and Neuroadaptation

Symptoms displayed in a cocaine-abuser might indicate: preexistent psychopathology, a predisposition to psychiatric disorder that is unmasked or exacerbated by chronic cocaine use, or psychiatric sequelae that are a direct consequence of cocaine use. There are no data available on whether or how often each of these exist in cocaine abusing populations. Such data are crucial to sample comparability. Further, there is no longitudinal data available to determine whether impairment increases with time. Does chronic cocaine create neuroadaptation and psychiatric disorder in humans? Exclusive of psychiatric diagnoses such as MDI or ADD, we have hypothesized that the cocaine-induced neuroadaptation observed in animals has a clinical parallel in a progressive dysphoric anhedonia—similar to the severity spectrum in atypical depression, or to the anhedonic spectrum of endogenomorphic depression (extending from subaffective dysthymic disorder, through dysthymic disorder, and to unipolar depression)—with the severity dependent on the degree and duration of exposure to cocaine and/or on genetically based vulnerability to cocaine neurotoxicity (Gawin & Kleber, 1985b and 1985d). Similarly, our clinical impression is that a reverse progression and recovery occurs with prolonged abstinence. There are as yet no data to indicate whether these are actual changeable stages in cocaine abuse and recovery, or are instead depressive disorders of varying severity that preceded cocaine abuse and provided a foundation for cocaine self-medication. Consequently, such issues as staging dysphoria (a concept related to abuse severity but one that focuses on symptom presentation and magnitude rather than degree of craving or dyscontrol over urges to use cocaine), and/or the presence and distribution of depressive disorders may be central to understanding research samples and the specificity of treatment effects. Unfortunately, a great deal of detailed descriptive and longitudinal study of cocaine abusers will be necessary before samples in treatment will be reasonably understood, and rational comparisons of treatment efficacy across studies will be possible.

CONCLUSIONS

There is no definitive knowledge available for any aspect of cocaine-abuse treatment. A number of approaches are in current use and a number of issues require resolution. Preliminary data on pharmacologic treatments are beginning to appear and pharmacologic adjuncts show much potential promise. However, it currently appears no more likely that any single treatment will arise as a definitive treatment for all cocaine abusers than it has for opiate abusers. Given that there are substantial areas in need of further research, it appears that current treatment for cocaine abusers should incorporate a flexible clinical integration of various approaches based on the characteristics, needs, and history of the individual patient.

REFERENCES

AMA Council on Scientific Affairs (1978) Clinical aspects of amphetamine abuse. *JAMA*, 240 (21): 3217–2319.

Anker, A.L., Crowley, T.J. (1982) Use of contingency in speciality clinics for cocaine abuse. *National Institute for Drug Abuse Research Monograph Series* 4:452–459.

Banerjee, S.P., Sharman, V.K., King-Cheung, L.S., Chanda, S.K., Riggs, S.J. (1979) Cocaine and d-amphetamine induce changes in central B-adrenoceptor sensitivity: Effects of acute and chronic drug treatment. *Brain Res.* 175:119–130.

Baxter, L.R. (1983) Desipramine in the treatment of hypersomnolence following abrupt cessation of cocaine use. *Am. J. Psychiat.* 140:1525–1526.

Borison, R.L., Histri, A., Klawans, H.L., Diamond, B.I. (1979) A new animal model for schizophrenia: Behavioral and receptor binding studies. In Usdin, E. (ed.), *Catecholamines: Basic and Clinical Frontiers.* New York: Pergamon Press.

Brown, W.A., Corriveau, P., Egert, M.H. (1978) Acute psychologic and neuroendocrine effects of dextroamphetamine and methylphenidate. *Psychopharmacol.* 58:189–195.

Bunney, W.E., Garland, B.L. (1983) Possible receptor effects of chronic lithium administration. *Neuropharmacol.* 22:367–373.

Bunney, W.E., Post, R.M., Anderson, A.E., Kopanda, R.T. (1977) A neuronal receptor sensitivity mechanism in affective illness (a review of evidence). *Commun. Psychopharmacol.* 1:393–405.

Byck, R. Views of cocaine. This volume, Chapter 1.

Chanda, S.K., Sharma, V.K., Banerjee, S.P. (1979)B-adrenoceptor sensitivity following psychotropic drug treatment. In Usdin E. (ed.), *Catecholamines: Basic and Clinical Frontiers.* New York: Pergamon Press.

Charney, D.S., Menkes, D.B., Heninger, G.R. (1981) Receptor sensitivity and the mechanism of action of antidepressant treatment. *Arch. Gen. Psychiat.* 38:1160–1180.

Connell, P.H. (1970) Some observation concerning amphetamine misuse: Its diagnosis, management, and treatment with special reference to research needs. In Wittenborn, J.R. et al. (ed.), *Drugs and Youth.* Springfield: Thomas.

Cronson, A.J., Flemenbaum, A. (1978) d-amphetamineAntagonism of cocaine highs by lithium. *Am. J. Psychiat.* 135:856–857.

Crowley, T. (1982) Quoted in "Reinforcing drug-free lifestyles," *ADAMHA News,* August 27, p. 3.

Ellinwood, E.H. (1977) Amphetamine and cocaine. In Jarvik, M.E. (ed.),

Psychopharmacology in the Practice in Medicine. New York: Appleton-Century-Crofts, pp. 467–476.

Fibiger, H.C., Phillips, A.G. (1981) Increased intracranial self-stimulation in rats after long-term administration of desipramine. *Science* 214:683–685.

Fraenkel, H.M., Breek-VerBeek, G.V., Abriek, A.J., VanRee, J.M. (1983) Desylycinamide-arginine-vasopression and ambulant methadone detoxification of heroin addicts. *Alcohol and Alcoholism* 18:331–5.

Gawin, F.H., Kleber, H.D. (1984) Cocaine abuse treatment: An open pilot trial with lithium and desipramine. *Arch. Gen. Psych.* 41:903–910.

Gawin, F.H., Kleber, H.D. (1985a) Cocaine Abuse: Patterns and Diagnostic Distinctions, *NIDA Research Monograph Series* (in press). 1985a.

Gawin, F.H., Kleber, H.D. (1985b) Abstinence symptomatology and psychiatric diagnosis in chronic cocaine abusers. *Arch. Gen. Psych.* (in press).

Gawin, F.H., Kleber, H.D. (1985c) Neuroendocrine findings in chronic cocaine abusers. A preliminary report. *Brit J. Psychiat.* (in press).

Gawin, F.H., Kleber, H.D. (1985d) Cocaine anheldonia: endogenomorphic and atypical depressive models. (Submitted. 1985d.

Gold, M.S. (1983) 800 Cocaine/The first two weeks. Mimeographed report. Summit, N.J.: Fair Oaks Hospital.

Gold, M.S., Byck, R. (1978) Lithium, naloxone, endorphins, and opiate receptors: Possible relevance to pahthological and drug-induced manic-euphoric states in man. *The International Challenge of Drug Abuse.* National Institute of Drug Abuse Research Monograph Series 19 DHEW Pub. No. (ADM) 78–654. Washington, D.C.: U.S. Government Printing Office, pp. 192–209.

Gold, M.S., Pottash, A.L.C., Annitto, W.D., et al. (1983) Cocaine Withdrawal: Efficacy of tyrosine. Presented at the Society for Neuroscience, 13th Annual Meeting, Boston, November 7.

Goldberg, S.R., Spellman, R.D., Kelleher, R.T. (1979) Enhancement of drug seeking behavior by environmental stimuli associated with cocaine or morphine injections. *Neuropharmacol.* 18:1015–1017.

Helfrich, A.A., Crowley, T.J., Atkinson, C.A. (1983) A clinical profile of 136 cocaine abusers. *National Institute of Drug Abuse Research Monograph Series,* 43:343–350.

Khantzian, E.J. (1983) Cocaine dependence, an extreme case and marked improvement with methylphenidate treatment. *Am. J. Psychiat.* 140:784–785.

Kleber, H.D., Gawin, F.H. (1984) Cocaine abuse: A review of current and experimental treatments. *NIDA Research Monograph Series* 50:111–129. 1984.

Koide, T., Matshushita, H. (1981) An enhanced sensitivity of muscarinic cholinergic receptors associated with dopaminergic receptor sub-sensitivity after chronic antidepressant treatment. *Life Sci.* 28:1139.

Kokkinidis, L., Zacharko, R.M., Predy, P.A. (1980) Post-amphetamine depression of self-stimulation responding from the substantia nigra; reversal by tricyclic antidepressants. *Pharmacol. Biochem. Behav.* 13:379–383.

Kramer, J.C., Fischman, V.S., Littlefield, D.C. (1967) Amphetamine abuse patterns and effects of high doses taken intravenously. *JAMA,* 201:305–309.

Maddux, J.F., Desmond, D.P. (1982) Residence relocation inhibits opiate dependence. *Arch. Gen. Psychiat.* 39:1313–1317.

Maggi, A., U. Prichard, D.C., Enna, S.J. (1980) Differential effects of antidepressant treatment on brain monoaminergic receptors. *Eur. J. Pharmacol.* 61:91–98.

Mandell, A.J., Knapp, S. (1976)Neurobiological antagonism of cocaine by lithium. In Ellinwood, E.H. and Kilby, M.M. (eds.), *Cocaine and Other Stimulants.* New York: Plenum, pp. 187–200.

Naber, D., Wirz-Justive, A., Kutka, M.S., Wehr, T.A. (1980) Dopamine receptor binding in rat striatum: Ultradian rhythm and its modification by chronic imipramine. *Psychopharmacol.* 68:1–5.

Pert, A.C., Rosenblatt, J., Squillace, K.M., Post, R.M. (1979) Unpublished manuscript, 1979, cited in Post, R.M., Smith, S.S., Squillace, K.M., Tallman, J.P. Effect of chronic cocaine on behavior and cyclic amp in cerebrospinal fluid of rhesus monkeys. *Comm. Psychopharm.* 3:143–152.

Rappolt, R.T., Gay, G.R., Inaba, D.S. (1977) Propranolol: A specific antagonist to cocaine. *Clin. Toxicol.* 10:265–271.

Resnick, R.B., Washton, A.M., LaPlaca, R.W., Stone-Washton, N. (1977) Lithium carbonate as a potentia treatment for compulsive cocaine use: A preliminary report. Presented at the Thirty-Second Annual Convention and Scientific Meeting of the Society of Biological Psychiatry, Toronto, Canada, April 28–May 1.

Rosecan, J.S. (1985a) The treatment of cocaine abuse with imipramine, L-tyrosine, and L-tryptophan: An open trial with 25 patients. Submitted.

Rosecan, J.S., Klein, D.F. (1985b) Imipramine blockage of cocaine euphoria with double-blind challenge. Submitted. Siegel, R.K. (1982) Cocaine smoking. *J. Psychoactive Drugs* 14:271–359.

Simpson, D. (1974) Depressed rates of self-stimulation following chronic amphetamine in the rat: Elevation of these depressed rates by desmethylimipramine. Paper presented at the Eastern Psychological Association, April 19.

Smith, D.E. (1984) Treatment and aftercare for cocaine dependency.

Presented at the Institute of Alcoholism and Drug Abuse Studies Conference on Cocaine: Problems and Solutions, Baltimore, January 25.

Spellman, R.D., Goldberg, S.R., Kellaher, R.T. (1977) Some effects of cocaine and two cocaine analogs on schedule-controlled behavior of squirrel monkeys. *J. Pharmacol. Exp. Ther.* 202:500–509.

Taylor, D.L., Ho, B.T., Fagan, J.D. (1979) Increased dopamine receptor binding in rat brain by repeated cocaine injection. *Comm. Psychopharm.* 3:137–142.

Tennant, F.S., Rawson, R.A. (1983) Cocaine and amphetamine dependence treated with desipramine. *National Institute of Drug Abuse Research Monograph Series* 43:351–355.

Tennant, F.S., Rawson, R.A. (1985) Double-blind comparison of desipramine and placebo in withdrawal from cocaine dependence. *NIDA Research Monograph Series* (in press).

Washton, A.M., Gold, M.S., Pottash, A.I.C. (1985) Cocaine abuse: Techniques of assessment, diagnosis and treatment. *Psychiatric Med.* (In press).

Weiss, R.D., Mirin, S.M., Michael, J.L. (1983) Psychopathology in chronic cocaine abusers. Paper presented at the 136th Annual Meeting of the American Psychiatric Association, New York, May 4.

Wikler, A. (1973) Dynamics of drug dependence: Implications of a conditioning theory for research and treatment. *Arch. Gen. Psychiat.* 28:611–616.

Wise, R.A. (1980) Direct action of cocaine on the brain: Mechanisms of complex behavior. In Jeri, F.R., (ed.), *Cocaine*, 1980. Lima: Pacific Press, pp. 21–28.

Wurmser, L. (1974) Psychoanalytic considerations of the etiology of compulsive drug use. *J. Amer. Psychoanal. Assoc.* 22:820–843.

7 | Clinical Issues in Cocaine Abuse

THOMAS J. CROWLEY

I HAD very little experience with abusers of cocaine until the late 1970s. But I did know two things about cocaine. First, the animal research literature (reviewed in this volume by Dr. Woods) showed that the drug was highly reinforcing in self-administration experiments. Second, I knew that clinicians saw very few cocaine abusers. Those few who did come in for treatment tended to drop out early; presumably they relapsed, finding the cocaine made them feel good more rapidly than did treatment.

Then, in rapid succession in 1979 a young nurse and a young dentist entered our programs seeking treatment for cocaine abuse. Based on the ideas that these patients were using a very reinforcing drug, that they had a high risk of relapse, and that there was a strong possibility of early drop-out from treatment, I set specific goals of getting the patients abstinent and holding them in treatment to sustain that abstinence.

CASE EXAMPLE

The dentist was a 28-year-old married white male in private practice. In dental school he had been a class officer and an outstanding student despite a troubled background with an alcoholic mother who arranged for the patient to be raised in a series of foster homes. But in college and dental school the patient had settled down and performed admirably. Then a friend gave him a large amount of high-grade cocaine. The doctor used the drug intranasally with others in a social setting, but gradually the use escalated. When the supply ran out, the doctor began diverting pharmaceutical cocaine to his own use.

193

After about one year he began injecting the drug intravenously; he said that there was no particular reason for this switch beyond curiousity. Like the monkeys described by Dr. Woods, this man now had a ready supply of a highly reinforcing drug, a means for parenteral administration, and no effective social controls on his use of the drug. The frequency and amount of use rapidly increased, until the doctor eventually was taking as many as 60 injections per day and as much as 45 grams per week of pharmaceutical cocaine. He lost about 20 pounds in weight, his wife left, and he experienced seizures on several occasions. His practice deteriorated because he frequently was unavailable.

When the patient entered our hospital he showed mild confusion, psychological depression, and profound psychomotor retardation. The dental licensing board, which had been investigating the case, suspended the doctor's license shortly after the admission.

I recommended a "contingency contract" to assure the licensing board that it would be safe for the patient to resume practice, and to reduce the risk of relapse while keeping the patient abstinent and in treatment for some time. I encouraged this dentist to write a letter to the licensing board, stating that he had relapsed to drug abuse and that he was surrendering his license. I suggested that he deposit that letter with me. I further recommended that, in a written contract, he direct me to collect frequent urine samples from him and to mail the letter at any time that a urine contained cocaine, or at any time that he failed to provide a scheduled sample. The patient chose to follow these recommendations, and his lawyer used this contract to convince the board to reinstate the dentist's license.

The contract remained in effect for 14 months, and the patient and his wife frequently participated in psychotherapy sessions. Urines and frequent clinical examinations showed that the dentist remained abstinent throughout that time. After termination of the contract he continued in intermittent "check-up" visits. In the twenty-second month after signing the contract he had a five-day relapse to heavy cocaine abuse. Based on reports from his colleagues, the licensing board again suspended his license for several months. It is now five years since he signed the initial contract and, except for that brief relapse, this patient has remained free of cocaine.

FACTORS PREDISPOSING TO COCAINE ABUSE

Older reviews emphasized individual psychopathology in the origin of substance abuse. "Most members of this group are emotionally immature, hostile, aggressive persons who take drugs in order to secure relief from inner tension. They have few healthy resources or interests and are motivated by immature drives for immediate goals. The addict-to-be finds in the drug a release from tension felt as a restless need for pleasurable or exotic sensations, the satisfaction of a longing for artificial elation or peace. Conscious discomfort is eliminated, repressed drives may be released, and responsibilities evaded. Another group consists of frankly neurotic persons with anxiety, obsessive, compulsive, or psychophysiologic symptoms which are relieved by the drugs. The third group consists of persons who in the course of physical illness have received drugs over an extended period and after the termination of the ailment have continued their use. However, probably all persons who acquire addiction in this manner have some fundamental emotional problem which caused them to continue the use of drugs beyond the period of medical need" (Noyes & Kolb, 1958).

This unrelieved emphasis on individual psychopathology as the principal contributor to substance abuse would suggest that the current epidemic of cocaine use reflects increasing psychopathology in the general population, especially among younger Americans, in the last ten years. That seems unlikely. A variety of other factors reviewed by Crowley and Rhine (1985) help to account for the increase in cocaine abuse.

Essential to the recent explosion of cocaine abuse are the drug's sudden availability and wide acceptance. Even in a group as young as high school seniors, 47% reported in 1982 that it would be "fairly easy" or "very easy" for them to obtaine cocaine, and 40% said that they had friends who used cocaine (Johnston et al., 1982). If one's friends have used a drug and report no adverse effects, if friends can show one how to obtain and use the drug, and if the drug is widely available, there is considerable likelihood that one will try the drug. The happenstance of a friend's gift of cocaine initiated the tragic series of events described above for the dentist, and ready availability through diversion from legitimate sources sustained his use.

Another predisposing factor is the potent pharmacological reinforcement produced by cocaine. This drug powerfully drives continued self-administration by animals (see Woods, this volume). Thus, for those who are introduced to the drug through its wide availability and acceptance in society, there will be some propensity to continue and accelerate the self-administration. Clinical experience suggests that drugs are more reinforcing by parenteral routes of administration; the dentist's dosing accelerated more rapidly after he switched to the intravenous route.

In addition to these sociological and pharmacological variables, personal factors cannot be discounted. Many studies show that a general tendency to take risks correlates strongly with a tendency to experiment with drugs. Persons with antisocial personalities, persons undergoing a general propensity to take risks because of a manic episode, youth displaying rebellion against family or authority, and others who take risks with their health and welfare are less likely to avoid the repeated use of risky drugs. Male sex also predisposes to cocaine abuse; in cocaine clinics male patients outnumber females about three to one (see below). A history of prior drug use also appears to contribute; previous and seemingly harmless experience with marijuana may have convinced many people that other illicit drugs could be used safely. Our dentist, a male who had been an angry, rebellious risk-taker as a youth, had an extensive history of marijuana use.

Genetic factors definitely enhance vulnerability to alcoholism. Although there are no rigorous data regarding cocaine, we frequently receive reports of parental alcoholism from cocaine-abusing patients, such as the dentist described above. It is interesting to speculate that a genetically transmitted propensity to abuse alcohol also might predispose to cocaine abuse.

Finally, an absence of immediate and effective social controls on one's drug use permits unimpeded escalation of cocaine dosing. For example, the dentist's wife for a long time did not condemn his drug use; instead, she participated in it. A high probability of detection and punishment for drug use clearly is associated with a reduction in drug use (Crowley, 1984a).

EPIDEMIOLOGY OF COCAINE ABUSE

This patient was a small part of a startling increase in cocaine use and abuse in the late 1970s. For a number of years the National

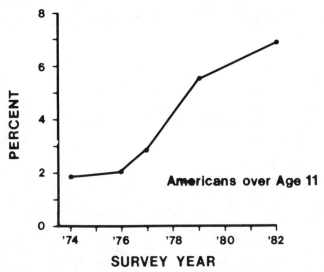

FIGURE 7.1. Percent of adult Americans who reported use of cocaine in the year preceding each survey in the NIDA Household Survey series (drawn from reference given in text.)

Institute on Drug Abuse has conducted household surveys, in which scientifically selected samples of the U.S. population are asked about their use of drugs. Figure 7.1, drawn from those data (National Institute on Drug Abuse, 1983), shows that the number of respondents who said that they had used cocaine within the preceding 12 months more than tripled between 1974 and 1982. And in both 1979 and 1982, about one-fifth of younger Americans reported cocaine use within the preceding 12 months (Fig. 7.2).

Regions apparently differed in extent of cocaine abuse. The number of emergency-room visits associated with the abuse of a particular drug is one way to assess the extent of that drug's abuse. By the early 1980s emergency-room visits for cocaine abuse were becoming common, and Denver ranked fourth in the country, far ahead of the national average but behind San Francisco, New York, and Miami in the proportion of cocaine-related emergency-visits (National Institute on Drug Abuse, 1982a). And in public drug-abuse programs, the percentage of cocaine-abusing patients was higher in Denver than in any other American city (National Institute on Drug Abuse, 1982b), so we were in a unique position to

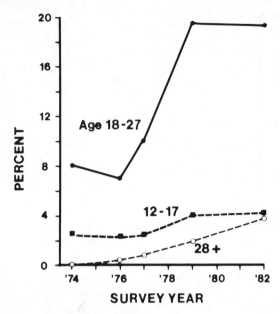

FIGURE 7.2. Percent of adult Americans (by age groups) who reported use of cocaine in the year preceding each survey in the NIDA Household Survey series (drawn from reference given in text).

examine the nature and course of cocaine abuse. Sadly, the rest of the nation apparently is catching up. Figure 7.3 shows the number of cocaine-related emergency room visits by annual quarters from 1981 to early 1984 nationwide (drawn from data in National Institute on Drug Abuse, 1984); visits have more than doubled in that period and the curve climbs steadily.

THE SIGNS AND SYMPTOMS OF COCAINE ABUSE

At the time that this epidemic of cocaine abuse was developing, Dr. Antoinette Anker Helfrich joined our group as a postdoctoral fellow. I encouraged her to describe this population of cocaine abusers, since descriptions of the condition were very scanty. And I recommended that she modify and apply contingency contracting techniques in an effort to hold patients in treatment, keeping them abstinent long enough to employ more traditional psychotherapeutic approaches.

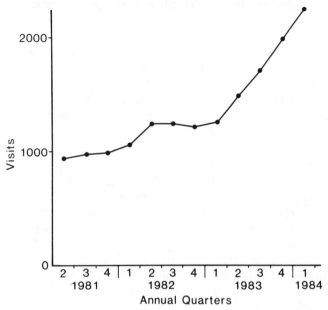

FIGURE 7.3. Cocaine-related visits to those hospital emergency rooms monitored by Drug Abuse Warning Network (DAWN; reference in text).

So Helfrich et al. (1983) described the signs and symptoms of 136 cocaine abusers who sought treatment in our clinics in Denver and Aspen. Over three-quarters of these patients who voluntarily presented for cocaine treatment were male. The mean age was 29 years. About one-fourth were married. Fifty-three percent ranked in the upper three of the five Hollingshead-Redlich social classes, and the group averaged 14 years of education; these latter figures were extraordinarily high for a public drug-abuse treatment program, emphasizing the difference between these patients and the more familiar "street" opioid abusers.

The patients reported a mean weekly dose of about 8 grams of cocaine (selling at $100 to $125 per gram). Fifty-seven percent used the drug intranasally, while 33% were intravenous injectors of cocaine and 10% smoked the free-base form of the drug. Seventy-two percent were using the drug several times weekly; nearly half used it several times daily. Unlike the "polydrug" abusers commonly seen in the 1960s, 40% of this group said that they concurrently were abusing no drug other than cocaine; 34% said that they concurrently were abusing only alcohol. Concurrent abuse of other drugs was uncommon.

Minor psychological problems, such as moderate depression, anxiety, irritability, guardedness, and suspiciousness were present in 99% of the patients. *Interpresonal problems*, including threatened or actual separations from loved ones or heightened discord in relationships, were reported by 87.5% of the patients. About 85% of patients complained of *financial problems* with diminished or exhausted resources or mounting debts. *Minor physicial problems*, such as weight loss, insomnia, dizziness, headaches, tremor, or nausea had been encountered by 81% of patients. Some 68% of patients had experienced *vocational problems* (job loss, impaired job functioning, absenteeism, supervisory reprimands, or loss of professional licensure or certification). *Major psychological problems*, including hallucinations, delusions, or serious suicidal thoughts or actions, troubled 43% of the patients. Such *major physical problems* as hepatitis, endocarditis, other serious infections, significant nasal bleeding or ulceration, loss of consciousness, seizures, and respiratory depression or failure, had occurred in 22% of patients. Only 15% of the group had experienced such *legal problems* as arrest, probation, parole, or investigation related to cocaine use.

The average patient had complaints in five of these eight symptom clusters, and among patients the number of problematic symptom clusters was highly correlated with the doses used. Not surprisingly, the more cocaine a patient used, the more symptoms he developed. However, the number of problematic symptoms was very weakly correlated with route of administration; the number of symptoms was a function of dose, but the route by which the drug was taken (intranasal, intravenous, "free-base" inhalation) apparently did not relate to the number of symptoms that developed. Contrary to popular opinion, cocaine by the intranasal route was not without hazard.

Although dose seems to be the main determinant of symptom severity, our clinical impression has been that patients who inject or smoke cocaine tend to escalate their doses more rapidly, arriving more quickly than intranasal users at problematic dose levels.

Of the 136 patients in that study, 76 completed Minnesota Multiphasic Personality Inventories (MMPI's). Dose modestly correlated with MMPI evidence of rebelliousness, social alienation, unconventional thinking, and resentment. The MMPI's usually were completed soon after the patient entered treatment, and we do not know whether the drug produced these MMPI changes, or whether preexistence of these personality characteristics had predisposed some patients to higher dosing.

Washton and Tatarsky (1984) provided cocaine information to abusers who phoned a "help line" in New York city. Interviews of the first 55 callers revealed clinical and demographic characteristics quite similar to those we had observed in Colorado. So it appears that cocaine abusers in different parts of the country share rather similar medical, psychological, and sociodemographic characteristics.

Considering these data together with other recent observations (Siegel, 1984; Washton & Gold, 1984; Cohen, 1984), we can define tentatively the pattern of signs and symptoms that result from progressive cocaine abuse. Some who try the drug once will experience an insidious increase in dose amount and frequency. This escalation probably occurs more rapidly among intravenous or pulmonary users. At present we only can speculate about what proportion of those who use cocaine will experience this gradual increase in dosing. As drug-related problems develop, some users successfully discontinue or reduce their dosing; others deny the nature or the extent of the problems and persist in escalating the dose. Eventually, most of those who seek treatment have sensed an inability to abstain from the drug without external assistance.

Certain specific signs and symptoms appear to result from actual, current *intoxication* with the drug. There is immediate post-dose physical or psychological pleasure, although patients commonly report a tolerance to the pleasurable effect of the drug. Psychomotor stimulation also follows a dose, but, again, patients report that extensive dosing produces tolerance to this effect. Tolerance to psychomotor stimulation among human patients is difficult to reconcile with the observed sensitization to motor stimulant effects of cocaine in experimental animals (see Post, this volume).

Patients report that as they take repeated doses of cocaine in a single dosing episode (e.g., during one evening), they develop guarded suspiciousness which may progress to frank paranoid delusions or hallucinations lasting a few hours to a few days. At higher doses (the required amount apparently varies among individuals) *acute overdose* phenomena may include muscle weakness and respiratory depression. Patients report that they become so weak after a large dose that they fall to the floor without losing consciousness, and feel unable to breath normally. Loss of consciousness and motor seizures also may occur. Respiratory depression and the musculature exertion of seizures may produce serious acidosis with associated cardiac arrhythmias. Resulting cardiac arrest is the apparent mechanism of death in severe overdoses. Because cocaine is rapidly metabolized, these overdose phenomena seem to peak within an hour following a large dose, resolving fully within a few hours.

In addition to these effects of acute intoxication, *chronic intoxication* may produce significant weight loss, a paranoid psychosis persisting for some days after termination of dosing, reversible organic mental confusion, profound psychomotor depression, and seriously impaired social and vocational functioning.

Abrupt cessation of dosing after many days of cocaine use does produce a mild *abstinence syndrome*, with symptoms opposite to the acute effects of the drug. Hypersomnolence appears; patients are fully arousable but are drowsy and sleep extensively. Vivid dreams, often with cocaine-related content, may occur. Hyperphagia develops; the patient described above gained 18 pounds in 18 days in our hospital. Psychological depression, with sad affect and crying is common. The hypersomnia and depression usually resolve within a few days, although heavy cocaine abusers often "awaken" to shattered life circumstances which may sustain dysphoria for many weeks or months. Overeating and cocaine-related dreams also may persist for many weeks to several months.

Finally, cocaine abusers may suffer from certain *medical problems related to the administration route.* Intranasal users commonly experience runny, stuffy noses, epistaxis, and nasal ulcers. Perforation of the nasal septum occurs, but fortunately is not common. Those who inject cocaine may develop abscesses at injection sites, systemic infections, bacterial endocarditis, or hepatitis. Any intravenous drug user risks Acquired Immune Deficiency Syndrome from needle-sharing, and limb death from accidental intra-arterial drug injections; there are as yet no case reports of these complications among cocaine abusers. Those who take the drug by pulmonary inhalation of cocaine fumes (free-base smoking) complain of sore throats and black or bloody sputum. Free-basing also may impair gaseous diffusion across pulmonary membranes (Weiss et al., 1981; Itkonen et al., 1984).

TREATMENT OF COCAINE OVERDOSE

Patients overdosing on cocaine often will have passed the acute crisis before arriving at an emergency room because of the drug's relatively short half-life (see Byck, this volume), especially if the drug was taken by a route assuring immediate absorption (intravenous or pulmonary). For those with persisting, serious toxicity, Gay (1982) recommended vigorous treatment, including, as needed, diazepam, thiopental, or succinylcholine for seizure control; propranolol for hypertension; lidocaine for cardiac arrhythmias, a cooling blanket for hyperthermia; and isoproterenol for catecholamine reversal. Gay suggested avoiding neuroleptic drugs, fearing reduction of seizure thresholds.

A recently reported case of cocaine overdose is informative because the patient was examined before, throughout, and after the episode (Jonsson et al., 1983). The patient was a "body-packer" who swallowed cocaine-laden condoms to smuggle the drug across national borders. He was arrested and hospitalized when X rays revealed the condoms in his gut. He passed most of them, and each contained about 20 gm of cocaine. The patient was given an enema to hasten passage of the remaining condoms, but one apparently broke, dumping perhaps 20 gm abruptly into his gut. Agitation, diaphoresis, and tachycardia developed suddenly, followed by a seizure, respiratory arrest, and hypotension. Blood pH plummeted to 6.83. Diazepam controlled the seizures, and artificial respiration with sodium bicarbonate corrected the acidosis. Cardiac arrhythmias which had developed with the acidosis soon resolved.

Recent studies of cocaine lethality in dogs (Catravas & Waters, 1981) and monkeys (Guinn et al., 1980) report mean lethal cocaine doses of 20 to 25 mg/kg. In both species chlorpromazine was an extremely effective antagonist of cocaine toxicity, and diazepam also reduced toxicity. Propranolol increased cocaine toxicity in both species.

Currently available information may suggest some revision of Gay's (1982) recommendations for treatment of cocaine overdose. The animal studies indicate that neuroleptics probably are beneficial, and that propranolol probably is harmful. The body-packer case emphasizes the importance of dealing vigorously with acidosis, and suggests that enemas are not helpful.

TREATMENT OF COCAINE ABUSE

The treatment of cocaine abuse is a growth industry. Many hospitals offer expensive in-patient treatment programs for cocaine abusers, and such treatment may be financially renumerative for treatment facilities. But how may one choose among the various treatments offered; which works best?

A controlled study of treatment outcome among substance-abusing patients requires, at least, random assignment of patients to different treatments, some objective measure of outcome, and some statistical comparison of outcome between treatment groups. At this writing no published study meets those elemental criteria, and I know of only one funded project that aims eventually to meet them.

Confronted with dangerously ill, desperate patients, and given no controlled studies of outcome, the best workers in this field necessarily are led to speculation and controversy. Excellent clinicians offer disparate recommendations: "The biochemical and neurophysiological deficits caused by cocaine-related hyperactivity should be treated by replacement therapy using precursors of neurotransmitters and vitamins" (Gold & Verebey, 1984). "Premature reentry into regular society should not be forced unless supportive therapy and exercise therapy have been initiated" (Siegel, 1984). In a maintenance model, as used with methadone, "methylphenidate might be useful in treating cocaine dependence because it ameliorates pre-existing or resultant behavioral and affective disturbances" and "might alleviate craving behavior and toxic-withdrawal symptoms" (Khantzian, 1983). When experienced experts in substance abuse offer treatment suggestions as divergent as vitamins, exercise therapy, and methylphenidate maintenance treatment, it is useful to review the evidence supporting various treatments.

Scott and Mullaly (1981) treated three cocaine-abusing patients who had persisting manic-like psychoses with lithium. All of the patients improved. Persisting manic-like psychoses, however, are not a common result of cocaine abuse. It is quite possible that these were manic-depressive patients whose manic indiscretions included excessive cocaine use. Thus, these cases may provide further confirmation for the use of lithium in the treatment of manic-depressive disease, rather than indications about lithium's efficacy in the treatment of cocaine abuse.

Anker and Crowley (1982) offered contingency contracts to 67 cocaine-abusing patients, the largest treatment series yet reported. The contracts, similar to the one described above, were accepted by about half of the patients. In the three-month follow-up there were very high rates of treatment retention and abstinence among those accepting the contracts, and very low rates among those who did not. Without random assignment to the two treatments, the authors note that the difference in the two groups could be due to preexisting motivation; the most motivated patients with the best prospects for successful outcome might have selected the rigorous contracting treatment. But the authors also discuss certain patterns in the data which suggest that differences between the treatments were more important in determining outcome than were preexisting characteristics of the patients. Although other uncontrolled clinical experiences (Resnick & Resnick, 1984; Horberg & Schnoll, 1983) also suggest some value in contingency contracting, final determination of this treatment's efficacy will have to come from controlled trials.

Khantzian (1983) reported treating one cocaine-abusing patient with the stimulant methylphenidate, in a daily maintenance regimen similar to methadone maintenance treatment for opiate addicts. This patient, who had been unresponsive to some other treatments, improved with one "isolated minor relapse" during a 20-week follow-up. Crowley (1984b) cautioned against widespread adoption of this treatment until further research demonstrated that uncontrolled methylphenidate abuse did not develop among methylphenidate-maintained patients.

Cocaine and the tricyclic antidepressants share some biochemical mechanisms of action, and depressive affect often follows termination of cocaine use. So there has been considerable interest in the possible treatment of cocaine abuse with antidepressants.

Baxter (1983) treated two patients who experienced marked hypersomnolence following termination of cocaine use. The hypersomnolence quickly abated after desipramine treatment began. Cocaine use in both patients apparently was unaffected by desipramine, for both patients quickly relapsed. And hypersomnolence *usually* abates within a few days after termination of cocaine use. So these cases provide little argument for tricyclic antidepressant treatment of cocaine abuse.

But Tennant and Rawson (1983) were more enthusiastic about desipramine treatment after their experience with 14 cocaine-abusing patients. Of the 14, 12 reported that desipramine reduced their craving for cocaine and their use of cocaine, although only 3 of the 14 continued desipramine treatment for more than one week.

Then Tennant and Tarver (1985) followed that original study (which had an open design) with the first controlled study of cocaine-abuse treatment. They randomly assigned 22 cocaine abusers to receive desipramine or placebo medication as outpatients, assessing outcome with such measures as duration in treatment, reported reductions in craving, sleep changes, and urinary evidence of abstinence. The patients remained in the study for a mean of 14 days. The only significant difference between the two groups was that placebo-treated patients reported sleeping better than desipramine-treated patients. So this study, with a classical double-blind design, found no value for desipramine in the early treatment of cocaine abuse.

Gawin and Kleber (1984) compared outcome in six desipramine-treated patients who wanted drug treatment vs. four patients who refused medication. There was a high rate of drug use among both groups in the early weeks of this three-month study, but all the desipramine-treated patients were reportedly abstinent during the last six weeks of the trial. Although encouraging, these results must be interpreted cautiously. The study was non-blind and the patients self-selected their treatments; it is possible (as noted above regarding the study of Anker and Crowley, 1982) that the less motivated patients chose the less rigorous, nonmedication treatment. There was infrequent urinary confirmation of self-reported abstinence. This also may have been an unusual group of patients, since all had remained in treatment with Dr. Gawin or elsewhere for at least four weeks before the study; patients dropping out from treatment at other clinics would not have "survived" long enough to be admitted into this research project. Finally, the "successful" patients in this study, who abstained in the final weeks of the project, would have been considered failures in the studies reviewed above because these patients used cocaine frequently in the early weeks of the project. So these interesting results suggest further research hypotheses but cannot confirm the merit of any treatment approach.

In the same report Gawin and Kleber (1984) examined outcome in six patients treated with lithium carbonate. Three reportedly remained abstinent throughout a three-month follow-up, while three others frequently used cocaine. It was reported that the abstainers shared certain characteristics of cyclothymic patients, while the nonabstainers did not. The meaning of these results is not entirely clear.

In the absence of well-substantiated protocols for treatment of cocaine abuse, my colleagues and I follow these guidelines in our Denver clinic. First, we require prepayment of a small fee before we set an appointment for an outpatient evaluation, and after that payment we see the patient as quickly as possible. We fear that an early relapse will cause patients to cancel even the first visit, and the commitment involved in prepayment, together with a very short waiting time, seem to get more patients to the first appointment.

At that appointment we evaluate the drug use (see Crowley & Rhine, 1985): what drugs were used, and when, where, how, with whom, and under what circumstances. We inquire about the perceived rewards of the drug use, and any experienced or feared adverse consequences. Unless the patient is psychotic, has serious medical problems, has an organic brain syndrome, is suicidal, lives in an environment that unambivalently supports continued drug use, or seems otherwise unable to participate in an outpatient evaluation, we set appointments for further evaluation over the next several days; fewer than 10 percent of our patients are hospitalized.

After a rapid but detailed evaluation we set treatment goals and describe contingency contracting, discussing possible contingencies with the patient. We offer frequent urinalyses, individual and couple or family outpatient therapy, and assistance in dealing with employers, legal agencies, and others with whom the patient's drug use may have produced conflicts. We encourage participation in Alcoholics Anonymous or Narcotics Anonymous. Given little evidence that medications are helpful, and believing that these patients need to find nonchemical means to solve life's problems, we rarely prescribe psychotropic drugs.

With those patients who choose to use contingency contracts, we agree on a consequence that the therapist will apply either if the patient's urine contains cocaine or its metabolite, benzoyl ecognine, or if the patient fails to produce a required sample. The patient directs the therapist to apply the consequence in a carefully drawn, written contract (see Crowley, 1984a). The patient then provides urine samples under observation each Monday, Wednesday, and Friday for one month. Thereafter, the patient calls for a recorded message each Monday, Wednesday, and Friday; on randomly selected days the message tells the patient to come to the clinic to provide a urine sample. Contracts usually are written to remain in effect for several months and usually sustain abstinence for that period. During that time we use traditional individual and couple psychotherapy, self-help groups, and relapse-prevention training to guide the patient toward continued abstinence from cocaine.

CONCLUSIONS

Cocaine is a highly reinforcing drug with a significant abuse liability when self-administered by any route. We certainly have not seen the last casualties from the current epidemic of cocaine abuse. An important public health priority should be to inform users and potential users of the serious adverse effects they risk through experimentation with cocaine.

The painful lack of controlled clinical studies of treatment out-come in cocaine abuse is not due to any dearth of excellent investigators in the field; the patients are very difficult to study. Patients often come to treatment desperate and in severe crisis, and they tend to drop out of treatment early. They often reject random-assignment protocols and research consent forms, feeling that their problem is too crucial to permit assignment to treatment on a random basis, and this attitude facilitates early drop-out from treatment research projects. Although research protocols may be arranged so that early drop-outs are discounted (e.g., only patients who remain in treatment for several weeks become candidates for research), such protocols beg a central clinical question: "How do we reduce drop-outs?" To be effective, a treatment for this condition should hold most patients long enough to secure abstinence, and a test of treatment efficacy should examine the treatment's ability to reduce drop-outs.

Clinical scientists who serve on grant review committees usually hew to strict standards of research design, including random assignment to concurrently treated groups. But a concurrent assign-ment protocol, described on a consent form presented early in a patient's contact with a clinic, may discourage the patient and facilitate early drop-out. Patients may accept random assignment to an active medication or a placebo, but in my experience they often drop out of treatment rather than risk random assignment among psychosocial treatments. One possible approach to this problem may be the use of nonconcurrent serial designs (e.g., all patients entering Research Clinic X during 1985 consent simply to receive treatment *A*, and all entering during 1986 consent to receive treatment *B*). Nonconcurrent serial designs raise certain problems, but the current absence of *any* controlled research on psychosocial treatments of cocaine abuse suggests that insistence upon perfect design may be preventing the accumulation of controlled data.

Finally, with cocaine abuse becoming a significant health problem, the American College of Neuropsychopharmacology and other scientific bodies are to be commended for their recent attention to the issue.

REFERENCES

Anker, A.L., Crowley, T.J. (1982) Use of contingency contracts in specialty clinics for cocaine abuse. In *Problems of drug dependence*, NIDA Research Monograph Series No. 41. Washington D.C.: U.S. Government Printing Office, pp. 452–459.

Baxter, L.R. (1983) Desipramine in the treatment of hypersomnolence following abrupt cessation of cocaine use. *Am. J. Psychiat.* 140:1525–1526.

Catravas, J.D., Waters, I.W. (1981) Acute cocaine intoxication in the conscious dog: studies on the mechanism of lethality. *J. Pharmacol. Exp. Ther.* 217:350–356.

Cohen, S. (1984) Cocaine: acute medical and psychiatric complications. *Psychiatr. Ann.* 14:747–749.

Crowley, T.J. (1984a) Contingency contracting treatment of drug-abusing physicians, nurses, and dentists. In *Behavioral intervention techniques in drug abuse treatment*, NIDA Research Monograph Series No. 46. Washington, D.C.: U.S. Government Printing Office, pp. 68–83.

Crowley, T.J. (1984b) Cautionary note on methylphenidate for cocaine dependence. *Am. J. Psychiat.* 141:327–328.

Crowley, T.J., Rhine, M. (1985) The substance use disorders. In Simons, R., Pardes, H. (eds.), *Understanding Human Behavior in Health and Illness*, 3rd edition. New York: William & Wilkins, pp. 730–746.

Gawin, F.H., Kleber, H.D. (1984) Cocaine abuse treatment: open pilot trial with desipramine and lithium carbonate. *Arch. Gen. Psychiat.* 41:903–909.

Gay, G.R. (1982) Clinical management of acute and chronic cocaine poisoning. *Ann. Emerg. Med.* 11:562–572.

Gold, M.S., Verebey, K. (1984) The psychopharmacology of cocaine. *Psychiatr. Ann.* 14:714–715;719–723.

Guinn, M.M., Bedford, J.A., Wilson, M.C. (1980) Antagonism of intravenous cocaine lethality in nonhuman primates. *Clin. Toxicol.* 16:499–508.

Helfrich, A.A., Crowley, T.J., Atkinson, C.A., Post, R.D. (1983) A clinical profile of 136 cocaine abusers. In *Problems of drug dependence, 1982*, NIDA Research Monograph Series No. 43. Washington, D.C.: U.S. Government Printing Office, pp. 343–350.

Horberg, L.K., Schnoll, S.H. (1983) Treatment of cocaine abuse. *Curr. Psychiatr. Ther.* 22: 177–187.

Itkonen, J., Schnoll, S., Glassroth, J. (1984) Pulmonary dysfunction in "freebase" cocaine users. *Arch. Intern. Med.* 144:2195–2197.

Johnston, L.D., Bachman, J.G., O'Malley, P.M. (1982) Student drug use, attitudes, and beliefs: national trends 1975–1982. NIDA. Washington, D.C.: U.S. Government Printing Office.

Jonsson, S., O'Meara, M., Young, J.B. (1983) Acute cocaine poisoning: importance of treating seizures and acidosis. *Am. J. Med.* 75:1061–1064.

Khantzian, E.J. (1983) An extreme case of cocaine dependence and marked improvement with methylphenidate treatment. *Am. J. Psychiat.* 140:784–785.

National Institute on Drug Abuse (September, 1984). DAWN Drug Alert. Available from Div. of Epidemiology and Statistical Analysis. NIDA, Rockville, Md.

National Institute on Drug Abuse (1983) NIDA capsules. Dept of Health and Human Services. Rockville, Md.

National Institute on Drug Abuse (1982a) Statistical series, annual data. Series I, No. 1, Dept. of Health and Human Services Publication (ADM) 82–1227. Rockville, Md.

National Institute on Drug Abuse (1982b) Statistical series, annual data. Series E, No. 25. Dept. of Health and Human Services Publication (ADM) 82–1223. Rockville, Md.

Noyes, A.P., Kolb, L.C. (1958) Drug addiction. In *Modern Clinical Psychiatry*, 5th Edition. Philadelphia, London: W.B. Saunders, Co., pp. 564–574.

Resnick, R.B., Resnick, E.B. (1984) Cocaine abuse and its treatment. *Psychiatr. Clin. North. Am.* 7:713–728.

Scott, M.E., Mullaly, R.W. (1981) Lithium therapy for cocaine-induced psychosis: a clinical perspective. *South. Med. J.* 74:1475–1477.

Siegel, R.K. (1984) Cocaine smoking disorders: diagnosis and treatment. *Psychiatr. Ann.* 14:728–732.

Tennant, F.S., Rawson, R.A. (1983) Cocaine and amphetamine dependence treated with desipramine. In Harris, L.S. (ed.), *Problems of drug dependence, 1982.* NIDA Research Monograph Series No. 43. Washington, D.C.: U.S. Government Printing Office, pp. 351–355.

Tennant, F.S., Tarver, A. (1985) Double blind comparison of desipramine and placebo in withdrawal from cocaine dependence. In Harris, L.S. (ed.), *Problems of drug dependence, 1984,* NIDA Research Monograph Series. Washington, D.C.: U.S. Government Printing Office, pp. 159–163.

Washton, A.M., Gold, M.S. (1984) Chronic cocaine abuse: evidence for adverse effects on health and functioning. *Psychiatr. Ann.* 14:733;737–739;743.

Washton, A.M., Tatarsky, A. (1984) Adverse effects of cocaine abuse. In *Problems of drug dependence, 1983.* NIDA Research Monograph Series No. 49. Washington, D.C.: U.S. Government Printing Office, pp. 247–254.

Weiss, R.D., Goldenheim, P.D., Mirin, S.M., Hales, C.A., Mendelson, J.H. (1981) Pulmonary dysfunction in cocaine smokers. *Am. J. Psychiat.* 138:1110–1112.

8 | Coca and Other Psychoactive Plants: Magico-Religious Roles in Primitive Societies of the New World

RICHARD EVANS SCHULTES

THIS CHAPTER is based on the keynote scientific address, entitled "New World Hallucinogenic Plants," delivered by the botanist Richard Evans Schultes at the annual meeting of the American College of Neuropsychopharmacology, on December 13, 1984, in San Juan, Puerto Rico.

The editors hope that its inclusion in this book will serve two major purposes. First: it lays out a comprehensive historical context regarding the varied roles of psychoactive substances derived primarily from plants in the cultures of the western hemisphere. This background provides an essential perspective for viewing our current range of multidisciplinary scientific interests in psychotropic drugs with "abuse potential," specifically cocaine, the central focus of this book. Second: this chapter, though perhaps admittedly insufficient from the botanist's viewpoint, brings to the members of the College a substantial body of information and additional sources for reading about many important psychoactive substances, which will serve as reference for those readers with a relatively slight acquaintance with the use of many of these compounds in primitive societies.

> Miracles . . . are performed throughout the world by these strange substances. . . . The savage in the jungle beneath a sheltering roof of leaves and the native of the storm-swept island secures through these drugs a greater intensity of life. . . . Not only are these drugs

of general interest to mankind as a whole, but they possess a high degree of scientific interest for the medical man, especially the psychologist and the alienist. . . .

> Louis Lewin, *Phantastica—*
> *Narcotic and Stimulating*
> *Drugs: Their Use and Abuse*
> *(1931)*

The use of narcotic, stimulant, and hallucinogenic drugs in primitive societies always and everywhere has been associated with religion, magic, and medicine. All three of these aspects are, for practical purposes, usually one part of a culture. This has been so since pre-history, and it is still true in our own times.

The hallucinogens, manipulated usually by the medicine-man, transport individuals from this mundane sphere to realms of ethereal wonder where, through hallucinations—especially visual and auditory ones—they can contact the spiritual forces that they believe cause all of mankind's woes, sickness, and death. Thus, the medicine-man believes that he can escape from the bonds of normal reality. Curiously, the drug addicts of our modern civilization, for a variety of reasons, similarly are attempting to escape from what they consider an oppressive reality. And when the physician administers chemical substances extracted from narcotic plants to lessen pain, he or she is helping the patient to escape the reality of pain. In my field work among aboriginal societies in the United States, Mexico, the northern Andes, and the Amazon, I have had always to attempt to view the use of hallucinogens and other psychoactive drugs as natural magico-medico-religious efforts to escape from what Norman Taylor has described as the "intolerable clutch of reality."

There are some 500,000 species of plants in today's flora of the world. Only a few of these species are psychoactive. Man in primitive societies feels the need to "explain" all phenomena. He explains the powerful, unworldly psychic effects of the psychoactive plants, especially the hallucinogens, by assuming that these few plants contain a resident spirit or divinity. Now, this is not too far removed from the usual Christian concept; one must only substitute a plant for the body of a human being.

As a scientist, I realize that the spiritual residents in these few plants are chemicals and that, in most cases, we can write these "spiritual forces" on the blackboard. Nevertheless, we should attempt sympathetically to understand the explanations prevalent in primitive societies around the world.

My principal interest in studying hallucinogenic drugs and identifying poorly known or unknown psychoactive plants has been centered—admittedly in a very limited way—on the possibilities of finding new chemical substances of vegetal origin that may be of service therapeutically or experimentally in modern medicine. Since I have worked primarily with psychoactive drugs of the New World, I am not considering the fewer but very important species used and valued in the Old World cultures.

When the Spanish Conquistadores, completely subservient to European culture and to the teachings of the Roman Church, arrived in Mexico, they were astonished that the Aztecs and other Indians worshipped their deities with the help of hallucinogenic plants. At that early period, the Europeans could not know that the strong psychic effects of these plants were due merely to chemicals, not to resident devils. Therefore, their persecution, initiated soon after Conquest, continued for several centuries and, in some circles, continues even today. We know much about the religious use of the psychoactive plants of that area and period, thanks to the often vitriolic reports concerning the dominance of these mind-altering drugs in native magico-religious ceremonies. These ceremonies have persisted in Mexico. We now know, furthermore, that many hundreds of years earlier there were sophisticated magico-religious ceremonies surrounding the use of psychoactive mushrooms in Guatemala, and archaeological finds dated as early as 1000 B.C. indicate the ceremonial use of the peyote cactus in southern Texas.

All of the sacred psychoactive plants in tropical America, except coca, continue to be used strictly as ceremonial magico-religious elements. Only the coca plant (*Erythroxylon* spp.) has become an hedonistically employed element—and even today there are indications that this plant has retained some vestige of its sacred role, as evidenced from certain beliefs about its origin and the almost ceremonial way in which it is cultivated and harvested, especially in the Amazon regions.

In aboriginal cultures, none of the numerous tropical American psychoactive plants, except coca, is misused or abused. The reason is clear: they are sacred elements, and the aboriginal society would not tolerate their abuse. Only in extremely isolated cases, where the traditional culture has broken down as a result of contact with Western civilization, has misuse or abuse been reported.

Because of the great importance of psychoactive plants in the life and traditions of several of our American aboriginal cultures, it may be significant to review briefly the botanical and chemical sources of some of these sacred elements of their societies.

CACTACEAE

Lophophora

By far the most important hallucinogen of pre-Conquest Mexico was the peyote cactus: *Lophophora Williamsii*. It may be called the prototype of New World hallucinogens because of its importance in primitive societies, its early attention from scientific investigators, and the isolation of an alkaloid—mescaline—that has been found to have value in psychological research and psychiatric treatment.

The genus *Lophophora* has two species: *L. Williamsii* and *L. diffusa*. The former grows in the dry, highland parts of central and northern Mexico and into Texas; the latter is known only from the Mexican state of Querétaro. *Lophophora diffusa* may not have been employed as an hallucinogenic agent, since its chemistry differs from that of *L. Williamsii* in almost lacking the vision-inducing alkaloid mescaline. Mescaline offered, for the first time, the possibility of studying visual hallucinations produced by a pure chemical compound. *Lophophora Williamsii* has 30% of its complex alkaloid content in the form of mescaline.

The ceremonial use of peyote apparently goes back several thousands of years. In a series of caves in Coahuila, Mexico, archaeological sites spanning about 8,000 years of intermittent occupation have yielded identifiable material, often in abundance, of *Lophophora Williamsii*, in association with remains of several other psychoactive or toxic plants (*Sophora secundiflora* and *Ungnadia speciosa*).

The earliest European reports hint that the Chichimecas and Toltecs knew peyote as early as 300 B.C.; although the accuracy of the dating may need rectification, the period is indeed early. The Spanish conquerors of Mexico, for the most part intolerant of pagan religious cults through repressive laws, diatribes, and persecution, tried to extirpate these "diabolic practices."

Sahagun* wrote in the late 16th century that those who eat peyote "see visions, either frightful or laughable; this intoxication lasts two or three days and then ceases; it . . . sustains them and gives them courage to fight and not feel fear nor hunger nor thirst; and they say that it protects them from all danger." He further reported that they "eat peyote, lose their senses, see visions of terrifying sights like the devil and were able to prophecy the future." He denounced peyote as embodying "satanic trickery."

In the same period, Hernández,** physician to the King of Spain, who spent five years studying Aztec medicines in the field, wrote in his great tome on medicinal plants, animals, and stones of "New Spain" that "both men and women are said to be harmed by it. . . . Ground up and applied to painful joints, it is said to give relief. Wonderful properties are attributed to this root [sic]. It causes those devouring it to be able to foresee and predict things . . . or to discern who has stolen from them some utensil." The Spanish effort to stamp out peyote went so far that, in 1760, a Catholic religious manual equated the eating of peyote to cannibalism.

In Mexico, the Huichols today journey annually for a peyote hunt to the deserts where the plant grows. It is ceremonially collected and dried for use throughout the year.

In the last century, Indians of the United States adopted peyote as a sacramental element in a new semi-Christian, semi-aboriginal cult; but the cactus was used in Texas as early as 1760 and was known to American Indians during the Civil War. After 1880, the new cult spread rapidly, spurred on by missionary activity on the part of Plains Indians. The speed of its expansion was due in part to the vision-seeking characteristics of many tribes but also in great part to the plant's reputation as a supernatural "medicine."

The cult encountered fierce opposition in the United States from Christian missionary groups, but eventually the Indians organized it legally as the Native American Church, which is said to have more than 250,000 adherents now in many tribes, even as far north as Canada. Their supplies of peyote are procured in the form of dried peyote crowns, known as mescal buttons, sent legally through the postal service.

*Sahagún, B. *Historia General de las Cosas de Nueva España*. Editorial Pedro Robledo, Mexico (1938).
**Hernández, F. *Nova Plantarium, Animalium et Mineralium Mexicanorum Historia*. B. Deuersini et Z. Masotti, Rome (1651).

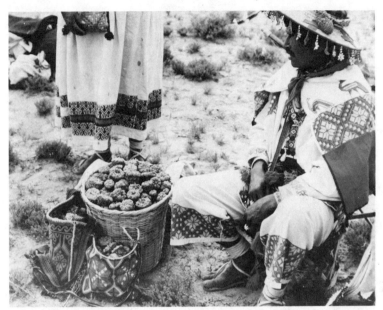

FIGURE 8.1. Huichol Indians ceremonially collecting peyote (*Lophophora Williamsii*). Chihuahua, Mexico. (Photograph: P.T. Furst)

The ceremony in the United States, though more or less standardized, varies somewhat from tribe to tribe. It consists of an all-night ritual, often in a teepee or special permanent building, with singing, chanting, meditation, prayer, and frequently a short "sermon" by the roadman or leader, ending in the morning with a communal meal. There is sometimes a healing ritual during the night.

Worshippers commonly consume as many as 30 or more mescal buttons during the night. The intoxication is characterized by a kaleidoscopically moving series of brilliantly colored visions. These visions are caused by one of the more than 30 alkaloids of two series (phenylethylamines and isoquinolines) contained in the plant—mescaline. Other hallucinations—especially auditory ones—are experienced during the intoxication, which tends to have two phases: a period of contentment and hypersensitivity followed by one of calm and muscular sluggishness, usually with hyper-cerebrality and visions. The visual hallucinations seem to follow a sequence from

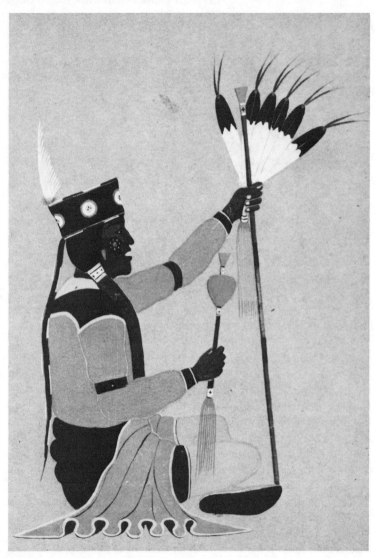

FIGURE 8.2. Kiowa Indian painting by Stephen Mopope of "roadman" or leader of Kiowa peyote ceremony, Oklahoma. (Original painting property of Botanical Museum of Harvard University)

geometric figures to familiar scenes and faces, to strange scenes and often a variety of unfamiliar objects.

When mescaline is employed in psychiatric research. The intoxication is induced by mescaline alone and is very different from that brought on by eating the mescal buttons with their more than 30 alkaloids, all or most of which are probably in some way physiologically active. There are no reports available about the individual biological activities of these minor alkaloidal constituents.

While the visions are usually important, especially among the Plains tribes where the vision-quest is deeply rooted, peyote is revered in great part because of its appeal as a "medicine" and stimulant. Peyote may have medicinal properties as understood in Western medicine, since antibiotic activity has been reported from the plant. Its supernatural "medicinal" powers, however, seem to stem from its bizarre visual hallucinations which, in native belief, are able to put individuals into contact with the spiritual realms from which come illness and death and to which the medicine-man may turn for diagnosis and treatment of many ills.

In Mexico especially, the magico-religious reputation of this cactus is so strong that many other plants are given the same or very similar names—not only numerous cacti but also species in other families, including the composites, legumes, orchids, nightshades, and others. It is the Cactaceae, however, that are, quite naturally, most closely associated in the Indian mind with Lophophora: species of Ariocarpus, Astrophytum, Aztekium, Coryphantha, Dolichothele, Echinocereus, Epithelantha, Mammillaria, Obregonia, and Pelicyphora. Most of these genera are known to be alkaloidal and potentially psychoactive, and they are associated aboriginally with Lophophora either because of some physical resemblance or because of their alleged or actual toxic effects.

Trichocereus

The San Pedro or aguacolla cactus, *Trichocereus Pachanoi*, or the central Andes of Bolivia, Ecuador, and Peru represents one of the hallucinogenic plants of most ancient use in South America. The oldest archeological evidence of its use is dated at 1300 B.C. Chavin textiles, almost equally as old, and ceramic vessels are decorated with the cactus together with the jaguar and humming birds. A whole series of archaeological records coming down to the Nazca culture from 100 B.C. to 500 A.D. depict the cactus.

When the Spaniards arrived, the use of Trichocereus in Peru was well established. The missionaries actively persecuted the San Pedro cult: "This is the plant," wrote one,* "with which the devil deceived the Indians . . . in their paganism, using it for their lies and superstitions . . . those who drink it lose consciousness and remain as if dead. . . . Transported by the drink,the Indians dreamed a thousand absurdities and believed them as if they were true."

The cult now practices an amalgam of pagan and Christian elements: the name San Pedro is believed to have been applied to the cactus because, like Saint Peter, it holds the keys to heaven. The rituals surrounding its use are heavily moon-oriented and are employed to "cure" a variety of ills from alcoholism to insanity; it is also valued in divination, to counteract witchcraft and sorcery. The magical powers of San Pedro transcend curing and divination: it is believed to be able to guard houses, for example, by whistling in an unearthly way, striking terror into the hearts of thieves and forcing them to flee.

Many patients with serious ailments make long pilgrimages to special shamans in holy places near lakes in the high mountains. Shamans distinguish four "kinds" of the cactus and identify them by the number of ribs. The plants with four ribs, very infrequently found, are considered to be endowed with the most potent supernatural powers.

Short pieces of the stem of *Trichocereus Pachanoi* are sold in native markets. They are boiled in water for as long as seven hours. The drink is often taken with the addition of other herbs, in which case it is known as cimora. Many of the additives—for example, the cactus *Neoraimondia marcrostibas, Isotoma longiflora, Pedilanthus tithymaloides*, and *Brugmansia aurea* or *B. sanguinea*—themselves may have highly psychoactive constituents. Frequently, magic calls for the addition of other elements, such as powdered bones and dust from graveyards.

Magical flight is typical of today's San Pedro ritual; Indians believe that they are carried across time and distance. The shaman may take the portion himself or with the patient. His aim is to make the patient "bloom" during the night ceremony so that his subconscious may "open like a flower," like that of the night-blooming San Pedro cactus.

*Sharon, D. *Wizard of the Four Winds*. The Free Press, New York (1978).

There are some 40 species of Trichocereus in South America; at least 25 are alkaloidal—some containing mescaline. *Trichocereus Pachanoi*, which occurs only at elevations between 6000 and 7500 feet, has a relatively high concentration of mescaline (2% of dried material) and some seven other alkaloids.

CONVOLVULACEAE

Ipomoea and *Turbina*

The early Spanish chroniclers of conquered Mexico wrote about the sacred seeds of a morning glory known as ololiuqui. They came from a vine with cordate leaves and small round black seeds called in Nahuatl coaxiluitl or "snake plant." For several centuries, the identity of ololiuqui was in doubt, notwithstanding excellent descriptions and illustrations of the plant in a variety of the early European writings. Identification had to wait until the early part of this century, and it was not until the 1930s that authentic botanical material collected among the Mazatecs of Oaxaca established beyond any doubt that the seeds are those of *Turbina corymbosa*, known formerly as *Rivea corymbosa*.

A second morning glory has recently been identified as an hallucinogen used among the Zapotecs of Oaxaca—the seeds of *Ipomoea violacea*, known locally as badoh negro.

Both of these morning glories owe their hallucinogenic activity to ergoline alkaloids. The seeds of both plants have very similar chemical contents, but the total alkaloid content of *Turbina corymbosa* is 0.012%, whereas *Ipomoea violacea* contains 0.06%, the reason for the natives' using in their ceremonies smaller quantities of seeds of the latter species than of the former.

A Spanish report* dating from 1615 stated that "it will not be wrong to refrain from telling where it [ololiuqui] grows, for it matters little that this plant be here described or that Spaniards be made acquainted with it." Another record of the same period** said that "when it is drunk, this seed deprives of his senses him who has taken it, for it is very powerful." Other references explained that

*Ximenez, F. *Quatro libros de la Naturaleza y Virtudes de las Plantas y Animales que estan receuidos en el Uso de Medicina en la Nueva España* . . . Mexico (1615).
**Ruiz de Alarcón, H. *Tratado de las Supersticiones y Costumbres . . . desta Nueva España.* An. Mus. Nac. Mexico 6 (1892), 134–137.

many things in Mexico (springs, rivers, mountains, ololiuqui, etc.) "have their deities. Ololiuqui . . . deprives those who use it of their reason. . . . The natives communicate in this way with the devil, for they usually talk when they become intoxicated with ololiuqui, and they are deceived by various hallucinations which they attribute to the deity which they say resides in the seeds."

A further report* said that "they place offerings to the seeds . . . in secret places so that the offerings are not found if a search be made. They also place these seeds amongst the idols of their ancestors. . . . They do not wish to offend ololiuqui with demonstrations before the judges of the use of the seeds and with public destruction of the seed by burning."

In Oaxaca, it is customary to grind the seeds of *Turbina corymbosa* on a metate. The resulting powder is soaked in cold water, which is strained through cloth and drunk. The ceremonial use of *Turbina corymbosa* is very common, at least in the hills of northeastern Oaxaca. Among the Zapotecs, the long angular black seeds must be collected by the person who is to take them. A young girl or boy must assist in the administration of the drink prepared from the seeds and must listen to the words uttered by the patient during his period of intoxication. The patient will, through the power of the seed of badoh, be enlightened as to the cause and cure of his problem; he will be told whether his trouble is actual illness or maliciously induced witchcraft. As one author** has written: "Today in almost all the villages of Oaxaca one finds the seeds still serving the natives as an ever present help in time of trouble."

There was little interest in *Turbina corymbosa* until the 1950s, when Humphrey Osmond's psychological paper appeared with the first report of experimental intoxication from the seeds, which the investigator had self-administered. The chemical constitution of these seeds was not clarified until the 1960s when Hofmann, the discoverer of LSD, elucidated the active principles of this morning glory. Prior to his work, no hallucinogenic compounds were known to exist in the whole morning glory family.

It has been suggested that the tlitliltzen of the ancient Aztecs was *Ipomoea violacea*.

*Serna, J. de la *Manual de Ministros de Indios para el Conocimiento de sus Idolatrias y Extirpación de Ellas*. Col. Doc. Ined. España 104 (1891) 163–165, Madrid.
**Wasson, R.G.: "Notes on the Present Status of Ololiuhqui and the other Hallucinogens of Mexico" in *Bot. Mus. Leafl.* Harvard Univ. 20 (1963), 161–163.

ERYTHROXYLACEAE

*Erythroxylon**

There can be no doubt that, with the exception of tobacco, the coca leaf represents the most important psychoactive plant of the New World. It is employed by millions of Indians in the Andes and western Amazon, and its main active alkaloid, cocaine, has long been a valuable asset in medicine and more recently has become a problem in a social abuse in Europe and the United States.

Archaeological materials of coca have been reported from the late Preceramic period along the dry Peruvian coast. Indication of the chewing of coca is found in the ceramic idols with distended cheeks—coquero figurines—found in Ecuador and dated about 1600 B.C., and earlier records can be found in the ceramic lime pots from the Valdivia culture dated approximately 2000 B.C. It is thought that coca has been used in Ecuador for 5000 years. Gold artifacts of coca chewers from Tiwanaku indicate the use of coca there perhaps as early as the fourth century A.D. There is a suggestion that the use of coca was introduced into Ecuador with the Inca conquest, but it is now certain that the chewing of these stimulant leaves is very ancient in Ecuador and that cultivation of the coca plant may have begun on the eastern slopes of the Ecuadorian or Peruvian Andes.

The chewing of the coca leaf may originally have been a closely guarded privilege of the Inca nobility and other officials, and that shortly before the Spanish conquest its use was extended to the general public, partly to increase work productivity. This belief has been questioned recently. It is true, however, that its use greatly increased following the conquest: many writers attest to the expansion of coca-chewing in daily life in the Andean region in the early colonial period.

The botany of *Erythroxylon* has only recently been adequately clarified, especially by Plowman and his colleagues: "Botanical studies on coca have redefined the earlier, simplistic view that coca

---

*According to the International Rules of Botanical Nomenclature, the correct orthography of the generic name should be *Erythroxylum*, even though the term is derived from Greek and not Latin. This has been elucidated by Plowman in *Taxon* 25 (1976), 141–144 and in *Botanical Museum Leaflets*, Harvard University 27 (1979),. 45–68. I prefer, nevertheless, to use the much more familiar and widely employed and etymologically more correct generic term *Erythroxylon*.

consisted of a single species—*E. Coca.*"* It is now recognized that two species and two varieties are involved. *Erythroxylon Coca* is wide-ranging, from Ecuador to Bolivia and northwest Argentina in the Andes; it occurs at 1500 to 6000 feet altitude in moist montane tropical forests on the eastern Andean slopes and in the wet inter-Andean valleys. *Erythroxylon Coca* still can be found wild in primary and secondary forests, and cultivated and wild populations freely interbreed. It differs from many cultivated plants in having been little changed in its morphology, genetics, and chemistry by cultivation.

Erythroxylon Coca var. Ipadu is a variety restricted to the western Amazon of Brazil, Colombia, Ecuador, and Peru. Some evidence suggests that it is a recent introduction, other evidence that its use is longstanding; but there is little doubt that the plant has evolved from the highland *E. Coca.* This variety is not known in the wild state.

A more drought-resistant type of coca evolved in the dry areas of northern Peru; it was described as *E. novogranatense var. truxillense.* It arrived early in the xerophytic parts of southern Ecuador and extended eventually southward in Peru and northward to the drier mountainous areas of Colombia, traveling even as far as Venezuela and, according to some reports, to Central America.

Erythroxylon novogranatense and its variety *truxillense*—the so-called Colombia and Trujillo coca, respectively—do not cross with *E. Coca* or cross with difficulty. It is postulated that *E. novogranatense* var. *truxillense* originated directly from *E. Coca* as an adaptation to drier conditions. It is further believed that *E. novogranatense* itself developed from the variety *truxillense;* it has a more northern distribution and is much more tolerant of ecological extremes. The earliest archaeological records of *E novogranatense* are dated to the first millennium A.D.

These several species and varieties vary in their chemical constitution, but all contain cocaine, the most significant psychoactive alkaloid of the genus. The alkaloids are of three basic types: derivatives of ecgonine, of tropine, and of hygrine.

The English plant explorer Spruce wrote over 125 years ago: "I could never make out that the habitual use of ipadú[coca] had any ill results on the Rio Negro [in the Amazon], but in Peru [i.e., in the highlands], its excessive use is said to seriously injure the coats of the

*Plowman, T.C. 1984 (see Selected References).

stomach, an effect probably owing to the lime taken along with it."* The German ethnologist Koch-Grünberg, the only other scientifically oriented researcher to have spent long periods in the western Amazon until recent years, wrote simply: "When used excessively, coca may be harmful to the nervous system."**

What is very commonly overlooked or even purposely ignored in many governmental and sociological circles is the fact that coca, as chewed by the native, is not of necessity physically, socially, and morally dangerous. Unwise legal prohibitions in certain Andean areas aimed at extirpation of the coca custom invariably have driven the Indian, deprived in his inhospitable, cold altitudes, of the stimulant and euphoriant coca, to the dangerously poisonous, badly distilled local alcoholic drinks, with an attendant rapid rise in crime of all kinds. Although coca-chewing may become habitual, true addiction, which in some cases may result from the use of pure cocaine, is not caused among the Indians who use coca leaves.

Coca is consumed daily in the highlands of Peru, Bolivia, the northwesternmost part of Argentina, and in parts of Colombia. The method of preparation and use varies little. The leaves are carefully dried. They are put into the mouth with an alkaline admixture, usually the ashes of quinoa (*Chenopodium Quinoa*), known as Peru as lliptu. Other sources of an alkaline admixture, which is necessary for the extraction of cocaine in the normally acidic mouth, are employed in regions where quinoa does not grow: lime itself may be used when available.

In the highlands, there is little vestige left of the sacred aura that once may have surrounded the plant. The leaves are chewed more or less habitually in daily life by people in many walks of life, especially by the Indians and many mestizos.

It is in the northwest Amazon that a semblance of sacredness survives—one of the reasons for believing that the coca custom may be of long standing in that region.

There are sundry substitutes for coca in the northwest Amazon. Probably a relatively large number of plants are involved, but only a few are known and have been definitely identified. The Boras and Witotos, for example, used two wild species of Erythroxylon when

*Spruce, R. [Ed. A.R. Wallace] *Notes of a Botanist on the Amazon and Andes.* Macmillan, london (1908). Reprinted ed., Johnson Reprint Corp. New York (1970).
**Koch-Grünberg, T. *Zwei Jahre unten den Indiamern.* Ernst Wasmuth A–G, Berlin (1909).

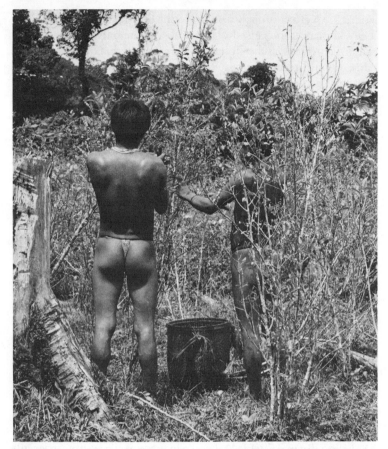

FIGURE 8.3. Makuna Indians gathering leaves of *Erythroxylon Coca* var. *Ipadu*. Río Piraparaná, Vaupés, Colombia. (Photograph: R. E. Schultes)

no cultivated coca is available. The Kubeos of the Colombian Vaupés may use *E. cataractarum*, a wild species, in place of real coca. Still other plant species may be substituted, although all are considered to be inferior to *E. Coca* var. *Ipadu*. In addition to their values as a narcotic, leaves of *E. Coca* var. *Ipadu* are used medicinally in the northwest Amazon for a variety of ailments.

Coca is prepared very differently for use in the Amazon than in the Andes. The leaves are carefully plucked each day by men, then toasted on a flat ceramic cassava-oven. When they are thoroughly dried and crisp, they are put into a large hollow trunk which serves

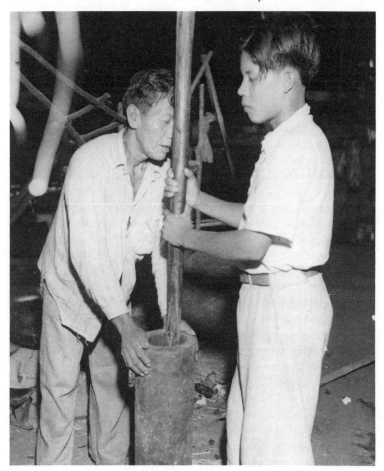

FIGURE 8.4. Kubeo men pounding toasted coca leaves in the mortar. Río Kuduyarí, Vaupés, Colombia. (Photograph: R. E. Schultes)

as a mortar and pounded to a powder with a large pestle of hard wood. The mortar measures four or five feet. The work of pulverization is done only by the men, who carry it out rigorously in a standing position. It may take up to a full hour of pounding. The dull, rhythmic thumping begins just at nightfall. In the meantime, leaves of *Cecropia sciadophylla* or, less frequently, other species of Cecropia or *Pourouma cecropiaefolia* are gathered and burned to ashes on the earthen floor of the Indian round house. The ashes are mixed with the coca powder in more or less equal quantity as an alkaline admixture. This mixture is then very finely sifted.

A number of other plants may be added as "flavorings." The most interesting additive is the smoke of the resin from a tree, *Protium heptaphyllum*, which the Tanimuka Indians blow into small piles of the coca powder; it lends an aromatic flavor to the powder.

The use of coca in the northwest Amazon is restricted to male members of the tribes. It is significant, too, that, while agriculture is the work of women, only men may tend the coca fields, which are always separate from the general agricultural plot. Intensity of use varies from individual to individual and from tribe to tribe. Although coca seems to have an essential and semi-sacred role in sundry ceremonies, it is employed hedonistically in daily life. Some Indians will take coca only in the afternoon or evening, but many keep the powder in the mouth throughout their waking hours. Some—especially among the Yukunas, one of the healthiest and most robust Indian tribes of the Colombian Amazon—consume huge amounts.

In regions where acculturation has not changed native custom, a visitor or stranger is made welcome with an offer of coca powder by the head of the round-house. A spatula made from the leg bone of the jaguar or a folded piece of the banana leaf are aboriginally used for transferring coca powder to the mouth, but now a metal spoon may be employed. A spoonful or two of the powder is put into the mouth; it is not chewed but is allowed gradually to mix with saliva and pass slowly into the stomach. When the dose is thus diminished, it is replenished with an additional amount. Normally, a "quid" is kept in the mouth throughout the day.

Coca is used in several other ways in the northwest Amazon. The Tukanoan Indians of the Río Papurí take an aromatic decoction of the coca leaf—whether for medicinal purposes or not is still not known. The Panabos of Amazonian Peru drink coca on occasion "to lighten the body." There are vague reports, still not verified, that the Yukunas and Tanimukas of the Río Miritiparaná utilize coca powder in certain ceremonies as a snuff; there is no pharmacological reason to presume that it could not be active when taken this way.

Erythroxylon Coca var. *Ipadu* is not only planted, collected, and treated in the northwest Amazon with particular respect, but the plant enjoys very special roles in certain ceremonies and even enters into the origin myths of the tribes. The Tukanoans say that the Sun

Father was a payé (medicine-man) who originated the knowledge and power of modern payés. He had in his naval the powder of vihó, the psychoactive snuff prepared from Virola. A daughter of the Master of Game Animals owned caapi, the psychoactive plant *Banisteriopsis Caapi*. Pregnant and in great pain, she lay down. An old woman, in an attempt to help, took hold of the girl's hand. The pregnant young woman broke her finger, but the elderly woman kept it and guarded it in the round-house. A youth, however, stole it and planted it. The caapi vine grew from this finger. Another daughter of the Master of Game Animals, also pregnant and in intense pain, lay down. An old woman came to help, but this time the woman seized the girl's hand and broke off a finger. She buried it. The finger took root and grew into the first coca plant.

Similar legends from many tribes of the northwest Amazon concerning the supernatural and ancient origin of *Erythroxylon Coca* var. *Ipadu* could be repeated; all bespeak great antiquity. Several tribes of the Colombian Vaupés, for example, say that their people originated from the Milky Way and arrived on earth in a canoe drawn by an anaconda. The canoe held a man and a woman, the cassava plant, *Manihot esculenta*, caapi and coca.

It is extraordinary that the history, botany, and ethnological studies of the use of one of the world's major psychoactive plants should have been neglected until very recent times. There is still much to be done in many fields impinging upon the aboriginal use of the species of Erythroxylon.

LEGUMINOSAE

Anadenanthera

A powerfully hallucinogenic snuff is prepared from the seeds of *Anadenanthera peregrina* (more widely known as *Piptadenia peregrina*) in northern South America, especially in the Orinoco basin, where it is called yopo. Apparently it was introduced and employed in pre-colonial times in much of the West Indies, where it was known as cohoba, but its use there has died out. The American ethnobotanist Safford identified the source of cohoba of the West Indies in 1916.

In the period of European conquest of South America, another psychotomimetic snuff was prepared in southern Peru, Bolivia, and

Argentina from *Anadenanthera colubrina*, where it was known variously as vilca, huilca, cébil, or sébil. This snuff is still employed by
Indians in the northern part of Argentina.

The active principles in both species are primarily tryptamine
derivatives and traces of beta-carbolines.

The earliest report of this snuff dates from observations made
among the Taino Indians of Hispaniola in 1496.* The observer
recorded that "these natives inhaled it to communicate with the
spirit world and that it was so strong that those who take it lose
consciousness; when the stupefying action begins to wane, the arms
and legs become loose, and the head droops . . . and almost
immediately they believe they see the room turn upside-down and
men walking with their heads downwards."*

The famous explorer of the Orinoco, Gumilla,** gave a graphic
account of yopo intoxication among the Otomac Indians in his book
El Orinoco Ilustrado, first published in 1741. "They have another
most evil habit of intoxicating themselves through the nostrils, with
certain malignant powders which they call yupa which quite takes
away their reason, and furious, they grasp their weapons. . . . They
prepare this powder from certain pods of the yupa . . . but the
powder itself has the odor of strong tobacco. That which they add
to it, through the ingenuity of the devil, is what causes the
intoxication and fury—they put their shells [large snails] into the fire
and burn them to quicklime . . . [which] they mix with the yupa . . .
and after reducing the whole to the finest powder, there results a
mixture of diabolical strength, so great that in touching this powder
with the tip of the finger, the most confirmed devotee of snuff
cannot accustom himself to it, for in simply putting his finger which
touched the yupa near to his nose he bursts forth into a whirlwind
of sneezes. The Saliva Indians and other tribes . . . also use the yupa,
but as they are gentle, benign and timid, they do not become
maddened like our Otomacos who . . . before a battle . . . would
throw themselves and, full of blood and rage, go forth to battle like
rabid tigers."

The British plant explorer Richard Spruce in 1854 gave the
earliest detailed report on the preparation and use of yopo snuff. He

---

*Bourne, E.G. *Columbus, Ramón Pane and the Beginnings of American Anthropology.*
Proc. Am. Anti. Soc. Worc. 17(1906)310–3–8.
**Gumilla, P.J. de *El Orinoco Ilustrado.* . . . 1(Ed. 1745)203–205, 305.

sent the pods and seeds for chemical study to the Royal Botanic Gardens at Kew, but the material was not analyzed until the 1970s. In these 120-year-old seeds, only bufotenine was found, whereas freshly collected seeds contained bufotenine with small amounts of N,N-dimethyltryptamine and 5-methoxy-N, N-dimethyltryptamine. Bufotenine is hallucinogenic, according to some investigators, although others have not been able to corroborate its psychoactivity.

MALPIGHIACEAE

Banisteriopsis

In the western and southwestern Amazon of Bolivia, Brazil, Colombia, Ecuador, and Peru and on the Pacific coastal region of Ecuador and Colombia, the Indians prepare a psychoactive drink from the bark of the malpighiaceous *Banisteriopsis Caapi*. The drink may be made exclusively of this species, but often other plants are added. More than twenty species are known as possible admixtures to the basic brew. The two most common plant additives are the leaves of the malpighiaceous *Diplopteris Cabrerana* (formerly known as *Banisteriopsis Rusbyana*) and the leaves of the rubiaceous *Psychotria viridis*.

The drink prepared only from the bark of *Banisteriopsis Caapi* is psychoactive; it contains the beta-carboline alkaloids harmine, harmaline, and tetrahydro-harmine. When the leaves of either the Diplopteris or the Psychotria are added, the intoxication is greatly lengthened and heightened; both contain tryptamines. Tryptamines are believed to have no psychotropic effects when ingested, unless in the presence of amine-oxidase inhibitors: the beta-carbolines are amine-oxidase inhibitors.

Several other malpighiaceous plants are reliably reported as the basis of hallucinogenic preparations, and they may well have similar chemical constitutions: two others are *Banisteriopsis muricata* and *Tetrapteris methystica*.

The drink prepared from the two species of Banisteriopsis is locally known as ayahuasca (Peru and Ecuador), caapi (Colombia and Brazil), pindé (the Pacific coast of Colombia), natema (Ecuador), or yajé (Colombia).

In his *Geografia del Ecuador*, published in 1858, Villavicencio identified the drug only as a vine employed by the Záparo and other

tribes of the Río Napo. He detailed its use to "foresee and to answer
. . . in difficult cases, be it to reply opportunely to ambassadors from
other tribes in a question of war; to decipher plans of the enemy . . .
and to take proper steps for attack and defense; to ascertain when a
relative is sick what sorcerer has put on the hex; to carry out a
friendly visit to other tribes; to welcome foreign travellers; or, at last,
to make sure of the love of their womenfolk."*

Seven years earlier, Spruce had found the Tukanoan peoples of
the Uaupés in Brazil using a liana called caapi to induce intoxication,
but his observations were published much later. He precisely
identified the liana as a new species of Banisteria, later known as
Banisteriopsis Caapi. Spruce even collected branches of the liana for
chemical analysis, but no analysis was made of them until 1969!
Again, when he entered the Ecuadorian Andes, he found the
Záparos using ayahuasca and deduced that it was identical with the
caapi that he had encountered in the Uaupés of Brazil.

Following Spruce's work, many writers, travellers, botanists, and
anthropologists have written about the drug, usually in a casual
vein, without helping to identify its botanical source. Outstanding
reports on anthropological aspects of the use of ayahuasca or caapi
come from Friedberg (1965) and Dobkin de Ríos (1972). Two
psychologically oriented studies—one in Ecuador and one in Colombia—are provided by Harner and Reichel-Dolmatoff, respectively.

The utilization and effects reported in various parts of the
Amazon differ widely. The Tukanoans of the Río Vaupés in
Colombia divide the effects of the drink into three stages: first,
vomiting, diarrhea, sweating, and a sense of flying through the air,
seeing at the same time brightly colored lights, soon to be replaced
by dancing, accompanied by a kaleidoscopic series of caapi-images
of a variety of geometric patterns. In the second stage, the geometric
figures disappear and are replaced by sensations of flight and
disappearance of space, accompanied by three-dimensional forms of
animals and monsters. The natives interpret these visions as validat-
ing their origin myths. This second stage characteristically contains
the deepest hallucinations, both visual and auditory: even singing
can be heard on occasion. The final stage is marked by brighter

*Villavicencio, M. *Geografía de la República del Ecuador.*R. Craigshead, New York
(1858).

Next, he snuffs, whilst, with the same reed, he absorbs the powder into each nostril successively. The hakúdufha obviously has a strongly stimulating effect, for immediately the witch-doctor begins singing and yelling wildly, all the while pitching the upper part of his body backwards and forwards."*

Botanical identification of several of the source species appeared in 1954; the use of two or three additional species has since then been reported.

In most of the northwest Amazon and Orinoco areas, the reddish resin-like exudate of the inner bark is prepared in the form of a snuff. In Colombia, the native medicine-men usually are the only members of the tribes to take the snuff. Among the Waikas of Brazil and adjacent Venezuela, however, all adult male members of the tribe may use the powder in ceremonies.The snuff as prepared by the Waikas from *Virola theiodora* appears to be much stronger than that of the Indians of Colombia. There are several variants in preparing the snuff, but the usual procedure involves scraping the soft inner layer of the bark and drying the shavings by gently toasting them over a fire; they are then stored until needed, when they are crushed and pulverized and triturated in a mortar and pestle made of a tropical fruit. The powder is sifted to a very fine, rich chocolate-brown, highly pungent dust. This dust is then mixed with an equal amount of the ashes of a leguminous tree, *Elizabetha princeps*. Occasionally, the aromatic leaves of *Justicia pectoralis* var. *stenophylla* are toasted and pulverized to be added to the snuff.

Among the Waikas, nyakwana snuff sometimes is taken hedonistically, but for the most part its use is ritual in ceremonies throughout the year. It is used to excess during the endocannibalistic ceremony of three or four days, during which the dead of the year before are memorialized. Shamans believe that with the help of the drug they can manipulate the friendly or enemy hikura spirits for good or even to kill people who live at great distances.

Instead of taking *Virola* in the form of snuff, the Witoto and Bora Indians of Colombia and Peru boil down an aqueous extract of the exudate to a thick paste which is rolled into small pellets. These pellets are then coated with a "salt"—the powdered residue from leached-out bark ashes from several plants. The pellets are then

*Koch-Grüberg, T. *Vom Roraima zum Orinoco*, Steker und Schroder, Stuttgart 3 (1923).

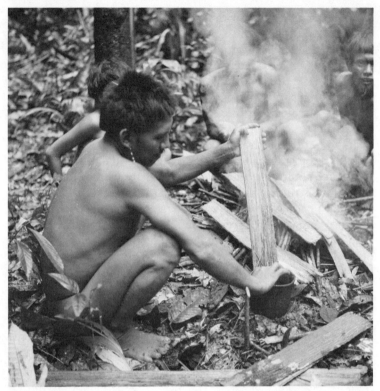

FIGURE 8.6. Waika Indian gathering the reddish resin-like exudate from the inner bark of *Virola theiodora*. Río Tototobí, Roraima, Brazil. (Photograph: R.E. Schultes)

swallowed or dissolved in water that is drunk. Intoxication begins in five minutes. More pellets may be taken to continue the effects.

One group of very primitive Makú Indians living along the Río Piraparaná in Columbia ingest the resin-like exudate crude, scraped from the bark with no other preparation.

The active principles of these species of *Virola* are tryptamines. The snuff made exclusively from *V. theiodora* by the Waika Indians along the Río Tototobí in Brazil contains 11% of several tryptamines, 8% of which is 5-methodxy-N,N-dimethyltryptamine. There is appreciable variation in alkaloid concentrations between different parts of the same plant.

In some species of *Virola*, small amounts of beta-carboline derivatives also have been found. They may act as monoamine oxidase

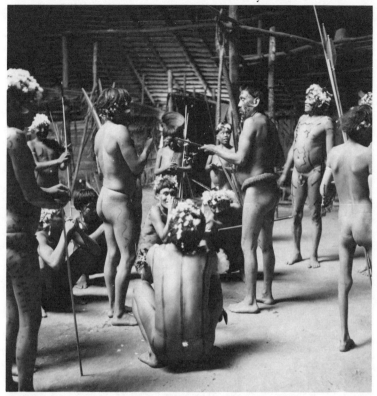

FIGURE 8.7. Waika Indians preparing to take nyakwana snuff. Río Tototobí, Roraima, Brazil. (Photograph: R. E. Schultes)

inhibitors, thus explaining perhaps the activity of *Virola* pellets when taken orally, since the tryptamines are believed not to be active when taken by mouth, unless in the presence of a monoamine oxidase inhibitor.

STROPHARIACEAE

Panaeolus, Psilocybe, Stropharia

In southern Mexico, some two dozen species of mushrooms are employed in magico-religious rites. They belong to several closely related genera: *Panaeolus, Psilocybe,* and *Stropharia.* All of the species have the same active alkaloids: psilocybine (an indole with a

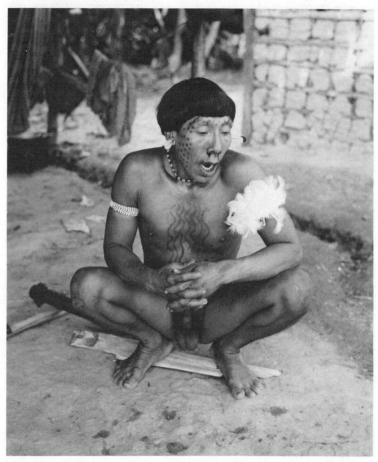

FIGURE 8.8. Waika medicine-man exhorting hikura spirits during ceremony in which nyakwana snuff is taken. Río Tototobí, Roraima, Brazil. (Photograph: R. E. Schultes)

phosphorylated hydroxyl radical, an acidic phosphoric acid ester of 4-hydroxydimethyltryptamine) and the rather unstable psilocine. It is of biochemical interest that psilocybine is substituted in the 4 position. Psilocybine has been used in psychiatry.

The ceremonial use of inebriating mushrooms existed in very ancient times. Frescoes from central Mexico, dating back to 300 A.D. have designs suggesting that worship of mushrooms occurred nearly two millennia ago. Even more remarkable and older are the artifacts called "mushroom stones," excavated in great numbers from highland Mayan sites in Guatemala. These effigies are variously dated but go back at least to 1000 B.C. They consist of an upright stem with a man- or animal-like figure crowned with an umbrella-shaped top.

We know much about the sacred use of mushrooms in post-Conquest times because the ecclesiastical authorities wrote so much about teonanacatl ("flesh of the gods") and even illustrated the fungi in various documents. A report written in the mid-1500s referred several times to mushrooms "which are harmful and intoxicate like wine" so that those who partake of them "see visions, feel a faintness of heart and are provoked to lust." Another reference* stated that the natives ate them with honey and "when they begin to be excited by them start dancing, singing, weeping. Some do not want to eat but sit down . . . and see themselves dying in a vision; others see themselves being eaten by a wild beast; others imagine that they are capturing prisoners of war, that they are rich, that they possess many slaves, that they had committed adultery and were to have their heads crushed for the offense . . . and when the drunken state has passed, they talk over amongst themselves the visions which they have seen."

One of the early Spanish ecclesiastical writings** was even more indignant. "They had another way of drunkenness that made them more cruel, and it was with some fungi or small mushrooms after them or eat with them a little bee's honey; and a while later they would see a thousand visions, especially serpents and as if they were out of their senses, it would seem to them that their legs and bodies were full of worms eating them alive, and thus half rabid they would sally forth from the house, wanting someone to kill them, and with this bestial drunkenness . . . it happened sometimes that they hanged themselves, and also against others they were crueler."

Another early observer recorded that inebriating mushrooms were part of the coronation feast of Montezuma in 1502. Hernández,*** who studied the medicinal lore of Mexican Indians for a number of years in the field, wrote of three kinds of mushrooms used as intoxicants and worshipped. Of some, called teyhuintli, he

---

*Sahagrin, loc. cit.
**Motilonia, T. de *Historia de los Indios de Nueva España.* Col. Doc. Historia de Mexico, Mexico (1858).
***Hernández, F., loc. cit.

explained that they "cause not death but madness that on occasion is lasting, of which the symptom is a kind of uncontrolled laughter . . . they are deep yellow, acrid and of a not displeasing freshness. There are others again which, without inducing laughter, bring before the eyes all sorts of things, such as wars and the likeness of demons. Yet others there are not less desired by princes for their festivals and banquets, and these fetch a high price. With night-long vigils are they sought, awesome and terrifying. This kind is tawny and somewhat acrid."

The Spanish authorities had been so successful in driving this cult into the hills that in more than four centuries anthropologists had not found a mushroom ceremony in Mexico. In 1915, the suggestion was made that, since dried mushrooms resemble the dried tops of the peyote cactus, teonanactl was merely another name for peyote—that both names referred to the same plant. It was suggested further that the Indians, to protect the sacred peyote, were pointing out mushrooms to fool the Spanish authorities. This misidentification of teonanactl was widely accepted, notwithstanding protests, until the 1930s, when identifiable specimens of *Panaeolus sphinctrinus* and another mushroon were collected with data on their use as hallucinogens by the Mazatecs of Oaxaca. The second mushroom was not botanically identified, until a number of years later when it was determined to be *Stropharia cubensis*.

In 1953, fortunately, the ethnomycologic team of R. Gordon Wasson and his wife, having read the earlier identification of *Panaeolus sphinctrinus* as an hallucinogen, began a series of well organized expeditions to various parts of Oaxaca. Sensing the need for interdisciplinary and intensive study of all aspects of the use of the mushrooms, Wasson enlisted the collaboration of sundry specialists—anthropologists, linguistic scholars, chemists, mycologists, musicologists, and others. As a result of this serious investigation and later studies by other mycologists, it is now known that some 25 species of mushrooms are ritualistically employed in southern Mexico.

A relatively large number of mushrooms are used as divinatory and ceremonial agents in modern Mexico, and probably at least as many were known to the ancient inhabitants of the Aztec empire. The species involved include among others: *Psilocybe mexicana; P. caerulescens* var. *mazatecorum; P. caerulescens* var. *nigripes; P. yungensis; P. mixaeensis; P. Hoogshagenii; P. aztecorum; P. muriercula; Stropharia cubensis; Conocybe siligineoides; Panaeolus sphinctrinus.*

Undoubtedly there were many tribes in ancient Mexico that employed teonanactl, but today we know that the sacred mushrooms are consumed by Mazatecs, Chinantecs, Chatinos, Zapotecs, Mixtecs, and Mijes, all of Oaxaca; by the Nahoas of Mexico; and possibly by the Tarascanas of Michoacan and the Otomis of Puebla.

Aside from the all-important hallucinogenic effects of these Mexican mushrooms, the most outstanding symptoms are muscular relaxation, flaccidity and mydriasis early in the intoxication, followed by a period of emotional disturbances such as extreme hilarity and difficulty in concentration. It is at this point that the visual and auditory hallucinations appear, eventually to be followed by lassitude and mental and physical depression, with serious alteration of time and space perception. One peculiarity of this state that promises to be of interest in experimental psychiatry is the isolation of the subject from the world around him. Without a loss of consciousness, he is rendered completely indifferent to his environment, which becomes unreal to him as his dream-like state becomes real.

The psychotomimetic effects following the ingestion of 32 dried specimens of *Psilocybe mexicana*, as described by the Swiss chemist Albert Hofmann*, are significant: "As I was perfectly well aware that my knowledge of the Mexican origin of the mushroom would lead me to imagine only Mexican scenery, I tried deliberately to look on my environment as I knew it normally. But all voluntary efforts to look at things in their customary forms and colors proved ineffective. Whether my eyes were closed or open, I saw only Mexican motifs and colors. When the doctor supervising the experiment bent over me to check my blood pressure, he was transformed into an Aztec priest, and I would not have been astonished if he had drawn an obsidian knife. In spite of the seriousness of the situation, it amused me to see how the Germanic face of my colleague had acquired a purely Indian expression. At the peak of the intoxication, about 1½ hours after ingestion of the mushrooms, the rush of interior pictures, mostly abstract motifs rapidly changing in shape and color, reached such an alarming degree that I feared that I would be torn into this whirlpool of form and color and would dissolve. After about six hours, the dream

---

*Hofmann, A. "Psychotomimetic Agents" in A. Burger [Ed.] *Chemical Constitution and Pharmacodynamic Action*. M. Dekker, New York. (Ed. 2, 1968),169–235.

came to an end. Subjectively, I had no idea how long this condition had lasted. I felt my return to everyday reality to be a happy return from a strange, fantastic but quite really experienced world into an old and familiar home."

Among the Mazatecs, the shaman often may be a woman. One of the most famous female shamans enacted the all-night mushroom velada for the first time to people of European or North American culture: it was a velada at which Wasson was present. The participants took their portions of mushrooms by 1 o'clock. Visions began twenty minutes later. No one slept until 4 in the morning. In Wasson's words, "it was as though my very soul had been scooped out of my body and transfered to a point floating in space. . . . Our bodies lay there while our souls soared . . . we were seeing visions . . . at first . . . geometric patterns, angular not circular, in richest colors. . . . Then the patterns grew into architectural structures . . . in richest magnificence extending beyond the reach of sight. . . . We were split in the very core of our being. On one level, space was annihilated for us. and we were travelling as fast as thought to our visionary worlds."*

"When the last candle was extinguished, the shaman began to moan, low at first, then louder. Then the humming stopped, and she began to articulate isolated syllables, each syllable consisting of a consonant followed by a vowel. The syllables came snapping out in rapid succession, spoken, not sung, usually almost ventriloquistically. After a time, the syllables coalesced into what we took for words [in Mazatec] and the Señora began to chant. The chanting continued intermittently all night." Brief passages from the shaman's chanting state the following:

> The law which is good
> Lawyer woman am I.
> Woman of paper work am I,
> I go to the sky,
> Woman who stops the world am I,
> Legendary woman who cures am I.
> Father Jesus Christ
> I am truly a woman of law,
> I am truly a woman of justice. . . .

*Wasson, R.G.

Woman of space am I,
Woman of day am I,
Woman of light am I.
No one frightens him
No one is two-faced to me. . . .

I give account to my Lord
And I give account to the judge,
And I give account to the government,
And I give account to the Father Jesus Christ,
And my mother princess, my patron mother,
Oh Jesus, Father Jesus Christ,
Woman of danger am I, woman of beauty am I . . .

"The chanting and the oracular utterance turned out to be only a part of what we were to witness . . . the Señora was either kneeling or standing before the alter table gesticulating. . . . Then much later, the Señora made her way to the open space . . . and embarked on a kind of dance that must have lasted for two hours or more."

There are specific characteristics of the ceremony or velada. (1) Mushrooms are usually taken fresh. (2) The velada is held in response to a request by a person needing to consult the mushrooms about a problem. A complicated diagnostic or curing ritual frequently takes place during the all-night ceremony. (3) Darkness and isolation are requisites to the velada. (4) One or two monitors who do not take the mushrooms must be present to listen to what is said. (5) Certain abstinences must be practiced preparatory to the ceremony.

The use of psychoactive mushrooms is not known today among any aboriginal group in South America. However, many archaeological anthropomorphic gold pectorals from the Sinú culture of Colombia have been interpreted as suggesting the ceremonial use of mushrooms. The earlier, more realistic artifacts have dome-like caps separated from the head by stipes, and appear extremely mushroom-like; later artifacts became rather stylized, the domes losing their stipes and becoming affixed to the head. These artifacts commonly have been called "telephone bell gods." They are dated roughly to between 500 and 600 A.D. It is perhaps significant that several species of *Psilocybe* containing the active principles have been collected in the region of northern Colombia where these Indians lived.

The Yurimagua Indians of the westernmost Amazon basin in

Peru were reported by Jesuit missionaries in the late 17th and early 18th centuries to be drinking a strongly intoxicating beverage prepared from a "tree fungus." *Psilocybe yungensis* has been suggested as the identification of this "tree fungus." Field work in this region, up to the present, has not disclosed any practice of this kind, but it represents a cultural trait little likely to disappear spontaneously without leaving a trace at least, and the region is still inhabited by many Indians in relatively primitive conditions of culture.

The Jesuits' report* states that "the Yurimaguas mix mushrooms that grow on fallen trees with a kind of reddish film that is found usually attached to rotting trunks. This film is very hot to the taste. No person who drinks this brew fails to fall under its effects after three draughts of it, since it is so strong or, more correctly, so toxic." If the fungus be truly *Psilocybe*, what, then, might this "reddish film" be?

EPILOGUE

In view of the pervasive importance of psychoactive plants and their products in human societies, it is appropriate to recall the worlds of Louis Lewin,** the famous toxicologist and one of the pioneers in the interdisciplinary study of those agents that he termed the phantasticants.

These substances have formed a bond of union between men of opposite hemispheres, the uncivilized and the civilized; they have forced passages which, once open, proved of use for other purposes; they have produced in ancient races characteristics which have endured to the present day, evidencing the marvellous degree of intercourse that existed between different peoples just as certainly and exactly as a chemist can judge the relations of two substances by the reactions.

SELECTED REFERENCES

A full bibliography would be very extensive and, in reality, is not necessary for a short survey of this kind. Detailed and more extensive

*Schultes, R.E. "The Search for New Natural Hallucinogens" in Lloydia 29 (1966),293–308.
**Lewin, L., loc. cit.

bibliographic notes can be found in many of the references cited below. The references are arranged by topics.

GENERAL REFERENCES

Cooke, M.C. (1860) *The Seven Sisters of Sleep*. London: James Blackwood.
Dobkin de Rios, M. (1984) *Hallucinogens: Cross-cultural Perspectives* Albuquerque: University of New Mexico Press.
Emboden, W.A., Jr. (1979) *Narcotic Plants*. New York: Macmillan.
Furst, P.T. (1976) *Hallucinogens and Culture*. San Francisco: Chandler & Sharp Publishers.
Furst, P.T. (ed.) (1972) *Flesh of the Gods*. New York: Praeger.
Grinspoon, L., Bakalar, J.B. (1979) *Psychedelic Drugs Reconsidered*. New York: Basic Books.
Hansen, H.A. (1978) *Heksens Urtegård*. Gyldendal: *The Witch's Garden*. [trans. M. Croft] Santa Cruz, Calif.: Unity Press-Michael Kesend.
Harner, M.J. (ed.) (1973) *Hallucinogens and Shamanism*. London: Oxford University Press.
Hartwich, C. (1911) *Die Menschlichen Genussmittel*. Chr. Herm., Tauchnitz., Leipzig.
LaBarre, W. (1972) Hallucinogens and the shamanic origins of religion. In Furst, 1972, loc. cit. 261–278.
Lewin, L. (1964) *Phantastica—Narcotic and Stimulating Drugs: Their Use and Abuse*. London: Routledge & Kegan Paul.
Schultes, R.E. (1965) Ein Halbes Jahrhundert Ethnobotanik amerikanischer Halluzinogene. *Planta Medica* 13 126–157.
Schultes, R.E. (1970) The New World Indians and their hallucinogenic plants. *Bull. Morris Arb.* 21:3–14.
Schultes, R.E. (1972) The utilization of hallucinogens in primitive societies—use, misuse or abuse? In W. Keup (ed.), *Drug Abuse: Current Concepts and Research*. Springfield, Ill.: 17–26.
Schultes, R.E. (1976) *Hallucinogenic Plants*. New York: Golden Press.
Schultes, R.E. (1979) Evolution of the identification of the major South American narcotic plants. *J. Psyched. Drugs* 11:119–134.
Schultes, R.E., Farnsworth, N.R. (1980) Ethnomedical, botanical and phytochemical aspects of natural hallucinogens. *Bot. Mus. Leafl.*, Harvard Univ. 28:123–214.
Schultes, R.E., Hofmann, A. (1979) *Plants of the Gods—Origins of Hallucinogenic Use*. New York: McGraw-Hill Book Co.
Schultes, R.E., Hofmann, A. (1980) *The Botany and Chemistry of Hallucinogens*. Springfield, Ill: Charles C Thomas.
Soderblom, N. (1968) *Rus och Religion*. Uppsala: Bokfenix.

Völger, G. (1981) *Rausch und Realität—Drogen im Kulturevergleich.* Rautenstrauch-Joest-Museums für Völkerkunde der Stadt Köln, Cologne. Vols. 1 and 2.

CACTACEAE (CACTUS FAMILY)

Anderson, E.F. (1980) *Peyote, The Divine Cactus.* Tucson: University of Arizona Press.
Bruhn, J.C., Bruhn, C. (1973) Alkaloids and ethnobotany of Mexican peyote cacti and related species. *Econ. Bot.* 27:241–251.
Bruhn, J.C., Holmstedt, B. (1974) Early peyote research. An interdisciplinay study. *Econ. Bot.* 28:353–390.
Klüver, H. (1928) *Mescal, the "Divine" Plant and its Psychological Effects.* London: Kegan Paul.
LaBarre, W. (1938) *The Peyote Cult.* New Haven: Yale University Press, Publ. Anthrop., No. 13.
LaBarre, W. (1960) Twenty Years of peyote studies. *Curr. Anthrop.* 1:45–60.
Rouhier, A. (1927) *La Plante qui Fait les Yeux Emerveillés—le Peyotl.* Gaston: Doin et Cie.
Schultes, R.E. Peyote and plants used in the peyote ceremony. *Bot. Mus. Leafl.*, Harvard Univ. 4:129–152.
Slotkin, J.S. (1956) *The Peyote Religion.* Glencoe, Ill.: Free Press.

CONVOLVULACEAE (MORNING-GLORY FAMILY)

Osmond, H. (1955) Ololiuqui: the Ancient Aztec Narcotic. . . . *J. Ment. Scie.* 101:526–237.
Schultes, R.E. (1941) *A Contribution to our Knowledge of Rivea corymbosa, the Narcotic Ololiuqui of the Aztecs.* Botanical Museum Harvard Univ., Cambridge.
Wasson, R.G. (1963) Notes on the present status of olouiqui and other hallucinogens of Mexico. *Bot Mus. Leafl.*, Harvard Univ. 20:161–193.

ERYTHROXYLACEAE (COCA FAMILY)

Antonil (1978) *Mama Coca.* London: Hassle Free Press.
Duke, J.A., Aulik, D., Plowman, T. (1975) Nutritional value of coca. *Bot. Mus. Leafl.*, Harvard Univ. 24:113–119.
Naranjo, P. (1974) El cocaismo entre los aborigenes de Sud America: su difusión y extinción en el Ecuador. *America Indigena* 34:605–628.
Plowman, T. (1979) Botanical perspectives on coca. *Psyched. Drugs* 11:103–117.

Plowman, T. (1979) The identity of Amazonian and Trujillo coca in *Bot. Mus. Leafl.*, Harvard Univ. 27:45–68.

Plowman, T. (1982) The identification of coca (Erythroxylum species): 1860–1910 in *J. Linn. Soc. Bot.* 84:329–353.

Plowman, T. (1984) The ethnobotany of coca (Erythroxylum spp.), Erythroxylaceae. In Prance, G.T. Kallunki, J.A. (eds), *Ethnobotany in the Neotropics.* New York: New York Botanical Garden.

Plowman, T. (1984) The origin, evolution and diffusion of coca (Erythroxylum spp.) in South and Central America. In Stone, D. (ed.), *Pre-Columbian Plant Migrations* in Papers of the Peabody Museum of Archaeology and Ethnology, Vol. 76 Harvard Univ., Cambridge.

Rury, R.P., Plowman, T. (1984) Morphological studies of archaeological and recent coca leaves (Erythroxylum spp., Erythroxylaceae). *Bot. Mus. Leafl.*, Harvard Univ. 29:297–341.

Schultes, R.E. (1957) A new method of coca preparation in the Colombian Amazon. *Bot. Mus. Leafl.*, Harvard Univ. 17:241–246.

Schultes, R.E. (1981) Coca in the northwest Amazon. *J. Ethnopharm.* 3:173–194.

LEGUMINOSAE (PULSE OR BEAN FAMILY)

Adovasio, J.M., Fry, G.F. (1976) Prehistoric psychotropic drug use in northeastern Mexico and trans-Pecos Texas. *Econ. Bot.* 30:94–96.

Altschul, S. von R. (1972) *The Genus Anadenanthera in Amerindian Cultures.* Botanical Museum Harvard Univ., Cambridge.

Campbell, T.N. (1958) Origin of the mescal bean cult. in *Am. Anthrop.* 60:156–160.

Merrill, W.L. (1977) *An Investigation of Ethnographic and Archaeological Specimens of Mescalbeans (Sophora secundiflora) in American Museums.* Technical Reports No. 6, Research Reports in Ethnobotany, Museum of Anthropology, Univ. of Michigan, Ann Arbor, Contrib. 1.

Safford, W.E. (1916) Identity of cohoba, the narcotic snuff of ancient Haiti. *J. Wash. Acad. Sci.* 6:548–562.

MALPIGHIACEAE (BARBADOS CHERRY FAMILY)

Dobkin de Ríos, M. (1972) *Visionary Vine.* San Francisco: Chandler Publishing Co.

Friedberg, C. (1965) Des Banisteriopsis Utilisés comme Drogue en Amérique de Sud. *J. Agric. Trop. Bot. Appl.* 12:403–437.

Harner, M.J. (Ed.) (1973) loc. cit.

Naranjo, P. (1970) *Ayahuasca: Religion y Medicina.* Editorial Universitaria, Quito (1970).

Reichel-Dolmatoff, G. (1978) *Beyond the Milky Way: Hallucinatory Imagery of the Tukano Indians.* Los Angeles: UCLA Latin American Centre Publications.

Rivier, L., Lindgren, J.-E. (1977) Ayahuasca—the South American hallucinogenic drink. An ethnobotanical and chemical investigation. *Econ. Bot.* 26:101–129.

Schultes, R.E. (1957) The identity of the malpighiaceous narcotics of America *Bot. Mus. Leafl.*, Harvard Univ. 18:1–56.

Schultes, R.E., Holmstedt, B., Lindgren, J.-E. (1969) De plantis toxicariis e Mundo Novo tropicale commentationes III. Phytochemical examination of Spruce's original collection of *Banisteriopsis Caapi. Bot. Mus. Leafl.*, Harvard Univ. 22.

Spruce, R. (A.R. Wallace, ed.) (1908) *Notes of a Botanist on the Amazon and Andes.* New York: Macmillan. (Reprinted. New York: Johnson Reprint Corp., 1970.)

MYRISTICACEAE (NUTMEG FAMILY)

Brewer-Carias, C., Steyermark, J.A. (1976) Hallucinogenic snuff drugs of the Yanomamo Caburiwe-Teri in the Caubauri River, Brazil. *Econ. Bot.* 30:57–66.

Schultes, R.E. (1954) A new narcotic snuff from the northwest Amazon. *Bot. Mus. Leafl.*, Harvard. 16:241–260.

Schultes, R.E. (1967) The botanical origins of South American snuffs. In Efron, D., Holmstedt, B. Kline, N.S. (eds), *Ethnopharmacologic Search for Psychoactive Drugs.* Washington, D.C.: U.S. Government Printing Office, Public Health Service Publ. 1645.

Schultes, R.E. (1969) De plantis toxicariis e Mundo Novo tropicale commentationes IV. Virola as an orally administered hallucinogen. *Bot. Mus. Leafl.*, Harvard Univ. 22:133–164.

Schultes, R.E., Swain, T., Plowman, T.C. (1978) De plantis toxicariis e Mundo Novo tropicale commentationes .XVII. Virola as an oral hallucinogen among the Boras of Peru. *Bot. Mus. Leafl.*, Harvard Univ. 25:250–272.

STROPHARIACEAE (STROPHARIA FAMILY)

Heim, R., Wasson, R.G. (1978) *Les Champignons Hallucinogènes du Mexique.* Paris: Museum National d'Histoire Naturelle.

Ott, J., Bigwood, J. (eds.) (1978) *Teonanacatl: Hallucinogenic Mushrooms of North America.* Seattle: Madona Publishers, Inc.

Schultes, R.E. (1939) Plantae Mexicanae II. The identification of teonanacatl, a narcotic Basidiomycete of the Aztecs. *Bot. Mus. Leafl.*, Harvard Univ. 7:37–54.

Singer, H. (1958) Mycological investigations on teonanacatl, the Mexican hallucinogenic mushroom. Part I. The history of teonanacatl, field work and culture work. *Mycologia* 50:239–261.

Wasson, R.G. (1980) *The Wondrous Mushroom: Mycolatry in Meso-america.* New York: McGraw-Hill Book Co.

Wasson, V.P., Wasson, R.G. (1957) *Mushrooms, Russia and History.* New York: Pantheon.

Subject Index